Health professionals are increasin
publish their research, apply for gra....,
with the media, present conference papers and contribute
articles to professional journals.

Writing well is an essential professional skill and writing to
publish is an important aspect of professional development.
But how do you get published? Where do you start? How do
you know if your writing is good enough and what can you
learn to make it better?

Effective Writing for Health Professionals is an invaluable
insider's guide to publishing within the health profession,
providing handy tips on:
• Getting started
• The writing process
• Winning habits of successful authors
• Promoting your work
• Author rights and responsibilities

Many would-be writers—students, administrators, clinicians,
managers and academics alike—are often intimidated at the
thought of writing. This book will help to overcome this
writing block and introduce aspiring authors to the world of
writing and publishing in a professional capacity.

Written by a best-selling academic author, *Effective Writing for
Health Professionals* provides insights and strategies for publishing designed for nurses, midwives and health professionals.

Megan-Jane Johnstone is Professor of Nursing and Director of
Research at RMIT University, Melbourne Australia. She is the
author of two leading works, *Bioethics: A Nursing Perspective
and Nursing and the Injustice of the Law*, has contributed extensively to international journals and served on editorial boards.

EFFECTIVE WRITING FOR HEALTH PROFESSIONALS

A PRACTICAL GUIDE TO GETTING PUBLISHED

MEGAN-JANE JOHNSTONE

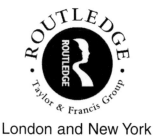

London and New York

First published 2004
by Routledge
11 New Fetter Lane, London EC4P 4EE
Simultaneously published in the USA and Canada
by Routledge
29 West 35th Street, New York, NY 10001
Simultaneously published in Australia and New Zealand
by Allen & Unwin
83 Alexander Street, Crows Nest, Sydney, NSW 2065, Australia
Routledge is an imprint of the Taylor & Francis Group

© 2004 Megan-Jane Johnstone

Typeset in 12/14pt AGaramond
by Midland Typesetters, Maryborough, Victoria
Printed by SRM Production Services Sdn Bhd, Malayasia

British Library Cataloguing in Publication Data
A catalogue record for this book is available from the British Library
Library of Congress Cataloging in Publication Data

ISBN 0-415-33447-0

To Arianthe and Margarita
for having the courage to follow your dreams

'when I ask you to write more books I am urging you to do what will be for your good and for the good of the world at large.'

—Virginia Woolf, *A Room of One's Own* (1945)

| CONTENTS

CONTENTS

| PREFACE

The idea to write this book and its compilation is a response to the many colleagues, associates and students who, over the past several years, have asked for advice on how they might begin a writing career and succeed as authors. Health professionals can make a difference to the world in which they live and work by writing and publishing their work in a range of media including professional journals, academic and professional texts, reports, professional newsletters and the mass-circulation media. Unfortuntely, many would-be writers in the health professions—clinicians, managers, administrators, academics and students alike—are often intimidated by the thought of writing and become their own instruments of discouragement. The primary aim of this book is to overturn this 'writing block' and to guide aspiring authors in the health care disciplines towards becoming their own mentors and instruments of encouragement and success.

In the chapters to follow I present information that will:

- assist readers to get focused on achieving their professional writing and publication goals
- demonstrate that writing is not just an intellectual event, but a craft, an art and science that can be learned and developed

- explore how writing and publication is not just about producing scholarly articles and texts, but about having a voice, naming a reality, touching an audience, developing professional self-understanding, advancing a cause and transforming the world in which health professionals live and work
- outline the processes for getting writing published
- facilitate readers on their journey and transformation from *writer* to *author*.

It is hoped that, upon reading this book, health professionals who have previously felt daunted by the prospect of writing will feel more confident about engaging in the writing process, get their work published, and will succeed as authors in their field.

| ACKNOWLEDGEMENTS

In writing this book, I have become indebted to a number of people. Foremost among these people are the many nurses, midwives and allied health professionals who have generously shared with me their stories of 'fears and failures' as aspiring authors and who have encouraged me to write this work. Their stories and aspirations have influenced significantly the nature and content of this book. Acknowledgement and thanks are also due to the publishing team at Allen & Unwin. In particular, thanks are due to Emma Sorensen (for her positive feedback and enthusiastic support of the work) and Cheryl Rose (for her meticulous editing of the manuscript and helpful comments).

1 | WRITING AND PUBLICATION IN THE HEALTH PROFESSIONS

Writing: the activity or skill of marking coherent words on paper and composing text (from Old English wrītan—originally: to scratch runes into bark).
— *The New Oxford Dictionary of English* (2001)

Publication: 1. the act or process of publishing a printed work. 2. any printed work offered for sale or distribution. 3. the act or an instance of making information public (from Latin pūblicāre to make public).
— *Collins English Dictionary* (1995)

Health professionals spend many hours (sometimes as much as 20 per cent) of their working day writing. This writing, largely undertaken for reasons of day-to-day professional communication, may take the form of responding to emails, compiling client case histories, annotating progress notes, writing letters and preparing various reports on a range of work-related matters. Some health professionals may also spend many hours writing outside of their usual work time, including writing entries in a reflective practice journal, composing an essay to meet the assessment requirements of a university course or preparing a presentation for a staff development seminar.

Despite the vast amounts of time that health professionals spend writing in the course of their work, few write specifically for the purposes of publication—even though publication in professional journals and texts can have enormous benefits and rewards. For many health professionals, the day-to-day demands of writing notes, compiling reports, and so on, is a burden and a chore. Thus any idea that writing for publication could be a pleasant and rewarding experience might appear, at best, to be far-fetched and at worse, misguided.

THE IMPORTANCE OF WRITING FOR PUBLICATION

There is no doubt that writing for publication and getting a manuscript published is hard work. Nonetheless publishing can be an extremely rewarding experience on both a personal and a professional level. On a personal level, getting a worked published can bring a great deal of personal satisfaction. On a professional level, the rewards of establishing a publication track record can include:

- professional development
- professional kudos and recognition
- career advancement.

In addition to the personal and professional rewards that can be gained by publishing professional works, there are other important professional reasons and imperatives for writing for publication.

Crucial to the development of any profession's unique body of knowledge and practice is the publication of its own distinctive professional scholarship. Further, it is vital that a profession's canon becomes well known to those both within and outside the profession, since this helps to facilitate both self and public scrutiny of the profession's knowledge and practice as well as the profession's responsibility and accountability to the public. Given these and related considerations, I believe that the issue of professional scholarship and publishing is an important one for members of the health professions.

THE GREATEST STORIES NEVER TOLD

Health professionals often have a wealth of knowledge and experience that deserves to be—and, as a matter of moral imperative, *ought* to be—'made public', in other words be *published*. This is especially so in cases where the publication of certain experiences and the knowledge gained from these experiences can provide valuable learning opportunities for others. Despite this, many health professionals (especially clinicians) do not write for publication or submit work for publication in a professional journal or text.

Several years ago I listened to an experienced intensive-care nurse give a heart-rending account of how she had dealt with an ethical dilemma in the intensive-care unit where she worked. Her story (prepared for and told as part of a formally assessed seminar presentation for a university course she was studying) involved the care of a man who was estranged from his identical twin brother whom he had not seen for several years. The man's condition was serious and it was evident that he was dying. Despite being aware of his deteriorating condition, the man was adamant that 'he did not want any contact with his twin brother' and that 'his twin brother was not to be contacted and told about his condition'. Having personally experienced the relationship dynamics between twins in her own family, and feeling intuitively that the man was not making the 'right choice' in the circumstances at hand, the nurse decided to respectfully disagree with her patient's request and to act against his expressed wishes. Recognising that time was running out (the man was not expected to live very long), she immediately set in motion a chain of events that resulted in the estranged brothers being happily reunited and reconciled before the ill brother died. Prior to the ill twin's death, both brothers were insistent that the nurse had done the right thing and expressed their deep appreciation for her insights, sensitivity and actions—especially her decision to go against the ill twin's expressed wishes.

The nurse's story provoked much controversy and discussion among those present at the seminar. Many were perplexed by the nurse's blatant, albeit considered, disregard of her patient's expressed wishes. Her audience recognised, however, that they had been privy to a unique learning experience and were unanimous in their response that the nurse should write up her story and get it published—not least because of the valuable learning it offered to others who might find themselves in a similar situation. The nurse responded shyly to this encouragement, stating only that she would think about it. Even though the views and counterviews expressed that day yielded all the ingredients for what promised to be a classic article on the ethics of respecting patients' choices, to this day the nurse has not published her story, or an analysis of it from a bioethics perspective. As a result, others have been deprived of a valuable learning experience. Why?

HURDLES TO PUBLISHING

The nurse's decision not to publish her story and the possible reasons influencing her decision are not unique. Indeed, there are many reasons why members of the health professions—especially clinicians—do not publish. For example, Paul Martin and Jay Birnbrauer (1996, p. 12), citing an early Australian survey of clinical psychologists reported that almost 62 per cent of respondents to the survey had never published a research paper in a journal and 83 per cent had never written a book chapter. The three most common reasons given for these low publication rates were found to be lack of:

- time
- research funding
- support by employers.

Nurses also have a low publication record. In one 1996 study by Kay Roberts, for example, it was reported that, of the nurses who publish, most were either senior nurse-academics or nurse-educators who hold post-graduate qualifications; and of these, most published in mainstream domestic (Australian) nursing journals. Even within this group, publication rates are poor. For instance, in 1997 the average publication rate for nurse-academics (who are expected to lead scholarship in nursing) was just under one per year, with refereed articles and book chapters accounting for only 25 per cent of scholarly output (Roberts 1997). A more recent study by Kay Roberts and Beverley Turnbull (2002/2003) has found that scholarly productivity in nursing has increased only slightly in the last five years. When it is considered that professors are expected to produce at least three or four peer reviewed publications per year, and lecturers at least one publication per year, it can be seen that there is considerable room for improving publication rates in the nursing profession. According to Roberts, the most common reasons cited by nurse-academics for their low scholarly output were lack of:

- time (exacerbated by teaching commitments and the need to get postgraduate qualifications)
- a research culture in nursing
- mentorship by senior nurse academics.

Publication rates for clinicians in nursing and midwifery are even lower than that of nurse/midwifery-academics (McConnell and Paech 1993). Common reasons for the low publication rate among clinicians are known anecdotally to include lack of:

- time
- employer support

- a research culture in clinical domains
- writing skills
- mentorship
- confidence (by prospective authors in their own ability to write and publish).

Poor publication rates and the hurdles to publication are not unique to psychologists and nurses, however. Other health professionals groups are also struggling to develop and sustain 'good' publication rates. Publication outcomes for clinicians in some areas of medicine, for instance, are relatively low. To cite just one example, Nicholas Wilson and George Thomson (1999) report that between 1987 and 1997, 91 registrars, who were training in New Zealand to become specialist public health physicians, produced 355 projects on public health and related issues. Significantly, only 28.5 per cent of these projects were associated with one or more publications that could be identified via literature searches using electronic databases, and of these only 17.5 per cent were published in peer-reviewed journals. Possible reasons for this poor publication conversation rate are not given.

Publishing outcomes among chiropractic faculty are also poor. In an award-winning paper on the subject, Dennis Marchiori et al. (1998), reporting on a survey administered to all full-time chiropractic faculty in the United States of America (n=972), found that the majority (72.2 per cent) of faculty members had not published a single peer-reviewed article in the last three years prior to the survey. Further, less than 2 per cent of the faculty members had published ten or more peer-reviewed articles in the last three years before the study. The report's authors concluded that 'the majority of publications are written by a minority of the faculty' and that this finding was consistent with other professions (including medicine and the allied health professions) (Marchiori et al. 1998). Barriers to publication were cited as including lack of:

- time
- technical support
- skills
- mentorship
- interest (Marchiori et al. 1998).

These examples demonstrate that the processes contributing to poor publication rates are a concern for all health professionals—academics as well as clinicians.

PUBLISHING FUTURES

In several respects the future of publishing in the health professions—especially among clinicians—may, at first glance, appear bleak. Clinicians continue to work in understaffed and high stress environments. At the end of the day they have little energy to *think* let alone write a reflective essay or commentary on a professional or practice issue. Furthermore, even those who work in academic institutions (and who are *expected* to publish as part of their specified work duties) find it difficult to meet the performance requirements of their roles, as the examples just given demonstrate. One undesirable consequence of this is that members of the health disciplines concerned are missing out on promotion opportunities, which, in turn, is leaving their disciplines under-represented and, hence, disadvantaged, at senior academic levels within the tertiary education sector. As Roberts (1996, p. 9) warns in relation to the nursing profession:

> Although the current rate of publication is understandable, it is not enough to ensure promotions for most of this group . . . Unless there is an improvement in the publication rate or a change in values in the higher education sector of the tertiary education system, an increased rate of promotion will be unlikely.

The status quo need not stand, however. It is possible—despite the constraints of work and time—to develop a strong publishing culture within the health professions. The question is: where do we begin?

A little over twenty years ago the *Australian Nurses Journal* (1982, p. 23) took the encouraging stance that writing was 'another professional dimension within the grasp of everyone' and challenged its readers with the following ideas:

> With writing we encounter a gift within the grasp of everyone, and this most serendipitous of discoveries comes about because writing is really only an extension of vocal expression. Which of us is incapable of 'speaking our minds', when the occasion arises? Which of us is incapable of writing something in the course of a nursing lifetime?

Health professionals are already deeply engaged in the processes of writing as a means of purposeful communication in the course of their day-to-day work. The challenge ahead is to extend this writing to a broader range of topics and a broader audience. To achieve this, however, a more 'futuristic' and proactive strategy is required. In particular, we need to make a steadfast commitment to the future of publishing in the health professions.

While we can't predict the future, we can, nevertheless, envisage a preferred future depicting our highest aspirations. We can also choose to shape our future according to these aspirations, as opposed to merely allowing ourselves to be at the mercy of outside forces and circumstances whereby we lose the capacity and energy to change and construct the world in which we desire to live and work. To succeed at this task, however, we need to change the way we think and work, and to *believe we can succeed* (Johnstone 2002).

In its *Guidebook for Nurse Futurists*, the International Council of Nurses (1999, p. 1) contends:

> Clarifying our aspirations for 'the future we want to create' is one of the most powerful ways of thinking about the future. The constant onrush of events and responsibilities diverts us from doing this kind of thinking. All of us need to pull back from our daily work now and then to reflect on what our aspirations really are and whether our major activities are really directed at pursuing those aspirations.

This view, originally aimed at nurse futurists and devised to encourage members of the nursing profession to think about the future of *nursing*, has equal relevance for our topic: *writing and publishing*. The future of publishing in the health professions rests on:

- clarifying our aspirations and goals as writers and authors in our chosen fields
- stepping back from the hustle and bustle of our daily routines to think about our future and where we want to be
- examining whether our decisions and actions are really directed at pursuing and achieving our publishing aspirations and goals
- recognising that while we cannot predict the future, we can, nevertheless, envisage a preferred future for publishing and can have a significant influence on shaping the future in which we will inevitably find ourselves
- believing that we can succeed.

SUMMARY

Writing is a core activity in the health professions. Nevertheless, few in these professions write *specifically* for the purpose of publication. There are many reasons for this situation, including but not limited to a lack of time, a lack of support from employers and peers, and a lack of confidence.

Over the years I have encountered many health professionals who have felt strongly about something, who have taken huge personal risks to engage in actions that have demonstrably helped others, who have discovered something during the course of their practice that is 'working' to the benefit of either their patients, their co-workers or their profession, and yet for a variety of reasons have neither written about nor published their experiences. This failure to publish and hence failure to share with others the knowledge and insights they have gained in relation to their experience results in lost knowledge and can have a profound impact on the lives of others—not least those dependent on them for care and/or service.

The primary objective of academic and professional writing is to make a significant and original contribution of knowledge to the field and to participate productively and influentially in professional conversations that have as their objective:

- questioning and calling into question 'things as they are'
- disseminating information and sharing knowledge that could improve policy and practice
- facilitating self and public scrutiny of a profession and its practice
- fostering professional accountability and responsibility to the public
- generally promoting the development of the discipline and the profession.

EXERCISES

1. Write down your professional goals and aspirations as a writer/author.
2. List what you perceive as being any obstacles to you achieving your writing/publication goals.
3. Outline what you believe would assist you to overcome the obstacles you have identified in question 2 (above).
4. Talk to a colleague or an associate who has had an article published in a peer-reviewed professional journal or who has had other works published. Ask them to tell you about their first experience of writing for publication. Ask what motivated them to write, how they got started and why they think publishing is important. Finally, ask them about what contribution they believe their work has made to their field/profession.
5. Talk to a colleague or an associate who has *not* published anything. Ask them to tell you why they have not published in a professional capacity and what if anything would motivate or assist them to write an article for publication in a professional journal.
6. Make a list of issues or ideas you think you would like to write about.
7. Imagine a preferred publishing future.

2 | GETTING STARTED

'The scariest moment is always just before you start. After that, things can only get better . . . if you are brave enough to start, you will.'

—King (2000, pp. 218–19)

'Every writer starts out as a beginner . . . All of us remain beginners no matter how much writing experience we may accumulate. After all, each time you start a new piece, you're bringing into existence something that hasn't existed before.'

—Edelstein (1999, p. 6)

Getting started can sometimes be an intimidating experience even for the most accomplished of writers. As one writer put it, 'The sight of a blank sheet of paper always intimated me; I felt too discouraged to even try more than a sentence or two' (Bryant 1999, p. 7). This writer eventually overcame the intimidation she felt at the sight of a blank sheet of paper and is now a successful author and seminar leader who has taught thousands of aspiring writers on the art, craft and science of writing.

Feeling intimidated by a blank sheet of paper—or a blank computer screen—and feeling daunted by the task of commencing a new work is entirely *normal* and more common than is admitted publicly. I certainly have experienced a fair share of feeling overwhelmed by the task of writing and of suffering the frustration of engaging in many false starts to a new work (on one occasion I made 40 attempts at writing the opening paragraph of a book chapter I was working on before I could proceed).

The key to overcoming this intimidation, and the frustration and discouragement that inevitably comes with it, is to:

- be clear about what your writing goals are and to focus persistently on achieving them
- get straight down to the business of choosing a topic, deciding your audience and selecting your publishing outlet
- commence the process of writing.

GETTING FOCUSED ON ACHIEVING YOUR WRITING GOALS

It is important that you clarify your writing aspirations and goals right at the outset of your writing career. This can be achieved by spending a few moments completing a simple self-assessment exercise that requires you to consider and note down:

- your mission as a writer
- your reasons for wanting to write
- what you most wish to achieve with your writing.

In completing your self-assessment and embarking on your writing career, it is important that you:

- set realistic publishing goals
- are path-orientated
- find a mentor to support you through your journey
- have a sense of your own 'voice'.

Different people will have different mission statements, different reasons for wanting to write, and different aspirations in regard to what precisely it is that they want to achieve with their writing. This difference is to be expected and should not be used as a measure for assessing the possible strengths and weaknesses of your own statements. What is important is that *you*, as an aspiring writer, are:

- clear about what it is you want to achieve
- determined to achieve your goals
- prepared to take the action and put in the effort necessary to realise your writing aspirations.

When I have facilitated seminars on 'Writing for publication', I have asked participants to identify the reasons behind their desire to write. The reasons given have ranged from being deeply personal to profoundly professional and/or passionately political in nature. Reasons commonly cited by seminar participants concerning why they want to write have included:

- to be visible
- so thoughts don't get lost

- to move on
- to prompt others
- to improve/advance ideas/others
- so others can read
- so others can be empowered
- I have something to say
- to find out what I know
- it feels good to order my thoughts on a [computer] screen
- for pleasure
- to alleviate pain/to heal
- to survive
- to make sense
- to inform
- to challenge
- to communicate with others
- to develop as a person
- to develop self-understanding
- to make a difference.

Those who write professionally and who have published extensively (both fiction and non-fiction writers) cite similar reasons for why they write (see, for example King 2000; hooks 1999; DeSalvo 1999; Blythe 1998).

Once you have clarified your mission as a writer, the reasons why you want to write and the goals you wish to achieve, there remains the tasks of choosing and confirming a topic, identifying your intended audience and choosing the best outlet for getting your work published. Often these things are decidedly simultaneously, but for the purposes of this discussion I will present them chronologically.

CHOOSING A TOPIC

Some of the richest sources of ideas and topics on which to write are your *own* observations and intuitions. Key issues and critical questions can be identified by:

- being observant
- looking for imperfections in things
- noting your own and others' dissatisfaction with things
- searching for causes
- being sensitive to implications
- recognising the opportunities embedded in controversy
- following your interest/curiosity—'following your passion' (Ruggiero 1995, p. 92; see also Seech 1997; van Hooft et al. 1995).

There are many examples of how personal observation, frustration and dissatisfaction, searching for causes and being sensitive to the implications of situations can yield rich material for writing professional articles. One such example can be found in the notable case of Olga Kanitsaki, AM, who is currently Professor of Transcultural Nursing and Head of Nursing and Midwifery at RMIT University in Melbourne. Kanitsaki first arrived in Australia in the 1960s as a non-English-speaking immigrant from Greece. She later trained and worked as a registered nurse in Melbourne. During the course of her work, Kanitsaki often observed patients of non-English-speaking and culturally diverse backgrounds being treated unfairly and in blatantly prejudicial, soul-destroying and harmful ways by attending health professionals of the day.

When interviewed in 1990 about her experiences, Kanitsaki, (1990, p. 16) recounted:

> There was a lot of prejudice. They used to say to me, 'Speak English', when I tried to help an elderly woman or man who couldn't speak English, by translating into Greek. The staff thought I was talking about them. I realised that there were reasons why people I worked with behaved the way they did. In order to understand their insecurities I had to ask how I could help them, rather than becoming defensive or angry about their behaviour.

Recognising the serious implications of cultural diversity in health care and the need for attending health professionals to be educated about these implications, Kanitsaki embarked on a twenty-year journey, writing and speaking about cross-cultural issues in health care (see various Kanitsaki in the bibliography, and Johnstone and Kanitsaki 1991). Her first article entitled 'Acculturation—a new dimension of nursing', published in the *Australian Nurses Journal* in 1983 and based on a clinical case study involving a Greek-born woman facing a leg amputation, is regarded today as a foundation article on the subject of transcultural nursing and health care. Today this article continues to be cited by other authors writing on the topic of transcultural health care and related issues. Her most recent work (Kanitsaki 2002) addresses the issue of culture, spirituality and mental health in the ethnic aged and draws critical attention to an area that has, up until now, been seriously neglected.

In 1995, Olga Kanitsaki was made a Member in the Order of Australia for her distinguished service to multicultural health care and to nursing. In 2000 she was awarded a Doctor of Philosophy from Melbourne University and was appointed as the first Professor of Transcultural Nursing in Australia. Kanitsaki's story is an outstanding example of how personal observations can lead to the writing of influential articles and to the development of an influential and distinguished writing and professional career.

Once you have chosen a topic, there are a number of other considerations that need to be taken into account. Specifically, you need to consider whether:

- you know the subject area well enough to be able write about it
- you feel strongly enough to write about it (for instance, do you have a real passion for the subject area?)
- anyone would seriously disagree with the position or viewpoint you are wishing to advance
- the topic is worth addressing at all (Seech 1997; van Hooft et al. 1995).

CHOOSING YOUR AUDIENCE

It is important to be clear right at the outset about *who* is your intended audience. Your intended audience can have an important bearing not only on *what* you write, but also on *how* you write it.

In deciding your audience, focused attention needs to be given to:

- identifying who, precisely, it is you want to inform (for example, is your target audience discipline-specific or multidiscipline in nature, novice or expert, gender-specific or gender-neutral, and so forth)
- deciding what it is you want to inform them about
- clarifying why you want to inform them (what are you trying to achieve by communicating your ideas and views to them)
- choosing the best medium to inform them (for example, choosing a specific journal, book or anthology).

CHOOSING YOUR PUBLICATION OUTLET

In choosing where to get your work published, remember that health professional groups constitute a niche market for commercial publishers. To put this simply, nurses, midwives, psychologists, occupational therapists, physio-therapists, chiropractors, medical practitioners and the like are recognised as small, specialised groups to whom those in the publishing industry can market journals and books profitably.

Professional niche markets provide aspiring writers (both novice and veteran) with extraordinary opportunities to publish. By virtue of their specialised knowledge, health professionals not only have a field to write in, but have a ready audience—and market—for whom they can write. In order to exploit this market well, however, prospective writers need to conduct some market research, in other words 'do their homework' to ascertain where the best and most appropriate opportunities lie. In particular, attention needs to be given to ascertaining:

- what's out there already
- who are the relevant editors or those who serve on the editorial boards of given journals
- what the editors are looking for
- what journals are appropriate
- which publishing companies are appropriate
- the prescribed word limits
- the styles that are used
- what topic to write about and how best to approach it (noting here a key maxim of publishing: 'Think outside the square' and ask yourself 'Can I approach this topic in a different way to others?').

Once you know what is out there—and what is wanted—it is much easier to pursue your publishing goals. Nevertheless, it is always important to be cautious in making your decision and to choose possible outlets for your work carefully. In making your final decision, consider whether a given outlet:

- will enable you to reach your intended audience
- will give you the scope you need in order to advance the discussion you wish to present, that is, in terms of:
  —specified word limit
  —editorial control
  —aims and objectives of the journal/publishing house
  —timelines
- is reputable (beware of disreputable or unscrupulous publishers that could be a disadvantage in the long term to your career or reputation).

Professional journals

Specialist professional journals constitute the main publishing outlet for health professionals and when embarking on a writing career, they are the best outlet for your first submission. Before submitting a manuscript to a professional journal for consideration, however, it is important to do two things:

- conduct an analysis of the journals available in your field to make sure you are choosing the most appropriate journal for your work
- ensure that you know and comply with the editorial requirements of the journal to which you have chosen to submit your manuscript.

Conducting an analysis of professional journals

As part of your analysis, you need first to survey the market to ascertain:

- which journals are publishing articles on topics relevant to your field of interest and/or expertise
- what makes each of the journals identified different from each other, for example:
  —who are the readers (will a given journal reach your intended audience)
  —what information are they seeking
  —what is being communicated
  —how widely is the journal being circulated/distributed
  —what are its publication standards
- whether the journal is indexed on relevant citation indexes; for example, the Cumulative Index to

Nursing and Allied Health Literature (CINAHL),
MEDLINE/PubMed.
*   the implications of submitting work to and having
    work published in the journal you are considering
*   the processes for submitting an article for review and
    publication in a particular journal
*   the editorial requirements of the journal.

Meeting editorial requirements

One of the surest ways of getting a manuscript rejected is
to violate the journal's editorial requirements. On one
occasion I had a manuscript rejected outright because of
my inadvertent failure to use American-English spelling
in just *one word*—which, unfortunately, happened to be
in the title of the manuscript! (I had spelt the word
'utilised' with an 's' instead of the American 'z'). The
manuscript was returned within a few days without being
reviewed. All that was attached to the returned manuscript was a photocopied section from what appeared to
be the journal's 'Guidelines for Authors' and on which
were highlighted in yellow the words emphasising the
imperatives of using 'American spelling'.

When preparing a manuscript for submission to a
professional journal it is essential that you obtain, know
and comply with the journal's editorial requirements,
which are usually contained in a section headed 'Notes to
contributors' or 'Information for authors'. This information usually appears on either the front or back cover of a
journal, or, in many instances, can be downloaded
from a designated Internet website (for example, the editorial requirements for professional journals published by

Blackwell Science can be obtained by visiting its website at <www.blackwell-science.com>).

Meeting the editorial requirements of a journal is a matter of common sense, but be aware, particularly, of the following:

1. *Editors*: approach in a professional manner (write formal letters accompanying submissions; use high-quality—preferably letter-headed paper, compose your letter carefully, and sign off formally).
2. *Manuscript*: submit required number of copies in the prescribed format (for example, A4 paper, double-spaced, single-sided, 3 cm margins, 50–100 word abstract, key words). Most journals give very specific instructions on how manuscripts should be submitted.
3. *Timelines*: know and meet timelines (develop a reputation for submitting on or before time). If your manuscript is accepted for publication on the condition that certain amendments are made, ensure that you make the required changes and get the amended manuscript back to the journal within the prescribed timelines. Failure to return an amended manuscript by the prescribed timeline may result in the work not being published. In the case of typeset proofs of an edited manuscript, if these are not returned within the time specified and no reason is given for the delay, they will generally be regarded as having been approved by the author and will be published as edited. If you are having difficulty meeting a deadline, write to the editor and request an extension of time.

4. *Word limit*: write to length (all journals are strict about prescribed word limits and some journals now require word counts to be provided).

5. *Style*: comply with prescribed referencing style; also comply with prescribed spelling requirements—for example, you may be required to use either English or American-English spelling.

6. *Submission integrity*: manuscripts are generally accepted on the understanding that the content has not been published or submitted elsewhere for publication; most journal guidelines carry a statement to this effect. It is usual practice that once you have submitted your manuscript you do not submit it elsewhere.

Academic publishers

Another (although less accessible) publishing outlet for health professionals is academic publishing companies. Sometimes the opportunity arises to contribute a chapter to a book being edited by another, or to write a book as a sole author or in collaboration with others.

As in the case of professional journals, before submitting a manuscript to an academic publishing house for consideration, you need to do some preparatory work, notably:

• survey the market for a prospective publisher
• initiate contact via a 'query letter'
• formulate a book proposal.

Market survey

As part of your analysis, you need first to survey the market to ascertain:

- which commercial publishers are publishing texts/ books on topics relevant to your field of interest and/or expertise. (To obtain this information, consult a local reference text of the kind which is usually published annually such as Rhonda Whitton's *The Australian Writer's Marketplace 2002: The complete guide to being published in Australia* or the UK *Writers' & Artists' Yearbook 2003* which provides information for authors in the UK and Ireland. These types of publishing guides can quickly become out of date, however, so make sure you check or buy the latest editions as they come out. Another way to assess the market is to review recent books published in the field and note who has published them.)
- what makes the various book publishers identified different from one another, for example:
  —who are the readers/what is the market being targeted
  —what information are they seeking
  —how successful are texts published by the company
  —what marketing resources do they have to promote the work
  —what is their overseas distribution
  —what is the commercial viability of the company
- what the implications are of submitting work to and having work published by the book publisher selected. For instance:
  —what are the restrictions on editorial freedom
  —what kind of copyright agreement is required
  —what editing standards will be applied
  —how do they deal with and relate to authors

—what provisions are included in the legal contract
—what royalties are paid (these can range from 7 to 15 per cent for academic texts, although author groups recommend that royalties should not be less than 10 per cent; Dunn 1999, p. 206).

- what the processes are for submitting a book proposal for consideration.

Query letters

Most commercial publishing houses will accept query letters about a book proposal. The aim is to generate interest in your work and to convince the acquisition editor that your proposal is a viable proposition. The general process you should follow in your approaches is:

- make sure you get the correct contact details of the acquisition editor
- avoid making contact by email
- telephone first, then follow up with a written response that includes a covering letter and your book proposal
- obtain a copy of the company's guidelines for submitting a book proposal
- write your covering letter in a professional manner and include a self-addressed envelope for a reply to or return of your proposal
- keep a record of the companies that you submit proposals to (including who you sent the manuscript to and when).

Formulating a book proposal

Most publishing companies have guidelines for prospective authors on how to structure and formulate a book proposal. Typically, publishers require:

1. *Information about the author*
   - Name, qualifications and professional affiliations.
   - Contact details: address, telephone and fax numbers (business and private), email address.
   - A brief description of your rationale for writing the book and your qualifications for doing so (if you have a successful record of publishing in professional journals this will enhance your credentials for writing a book).
2. *Information about the proposed book*
   - A complete book outline, including a brief synopsis of the content of each chapter.
   - The anticipated length of the manuscript and the proposed work plan and completion date.
   - Three representative sample chapters.
   - The primary (and secondary) market and the approximate numbers involved (e.g. how many readers).
   - The specific advantages your book will have over other competing works.
   - Reports on your other work.

In addition, publishers may require prospective authors to complete an 'Author marketing questionnaire' which they provide.

Newsletters and other print media

Another outlet for publishing work is a profession's or organisation's newsletter or newspaper (for example *Campus Review*). Being less formal in tone and format than peer-reviewed journals and texts, these outlets frequently provide a wonderful opportunity for aspiring writers to see their work 'in print'. Furthermore, editors of newsletters are *always* on the look out for material and often actively solicit contributions from associates in order to keep the publication viable.

I know of one nurse whose first publication consisted of an opinion piece on a professional issue that she wrote for *Nursing Review*, a monthly academic newspaper that has national distribution in Australia. Seeing her work in print gave this nurse an enormous boost in confidence and enabled her to progress to writing a more substantial work, which she eventually submitted, with success, for publication in a peer-reviewed professional journal. Inspired by this success, she is currently working on a second article for peer-reviewed publication.

Although contributions to newsletters and other print media are typically, and of necessity, smaller than those generally published in journals and texts, they neverthe-less require the same degree of focus, discipline and 'good writing' as their counterparts. In several respects they require *more* discipline on account of authors having to express their views in a concise number of words (often less than 500 words). Making an impact on readers in just 500 words is a challenge—even for veteran authors!

The key to writing a successful contribution for a newsletter or other print media is to write on a topic that is interesting and provide information that is useful to the stakeholders. In order to pitch your contribution at the right level, it is important that you clarify:

- who is producing the newsletter and for what purpose
- the aims and objectives of the newsletter
- who the readers are
- what they are reading for—that is, what are their interests, information needs and areas of concern
- how widely the newsletter is being circulated/distributed
- the circumstances under which constituents are likely to be reading the newsletter
- what, if any, implications there might be (good and bad) of you writing for the newsletter
- what the timelines for production are.

SUMMARY

Getting started on a new work can be an intimidating experience, even for the most experienced of writers. In order to overcome this 'block', it is important that you are clear about your writing goals and focus persistently on achieving them. Be very discerning in choosing a topic, deciding your audience and selecting your publishing outlet. You should also find a mentor—someone who can be a 'friendly critic' and who can support you on your writing journey. Once you have decided these things and have in place the necessary supports, you are then in a position to engage fully in the process of writing (the subject of the next chapter). This is where the real work begins.

EXERCISES

1. Complete the following statements:
   * My mission as a writer is to ....
   * My reasons for wanting to write are ....
   * What I most wish to achieve with my writing is ....

2. Compare your mission statement, reasons for wanting to write, and your stated writing aspirations with the statements of another aspiring writer and discuss the similarities and differences in your responses.

3. Drawing on your own personal observations and experience, identify a topic on which you would like to write an article.

4. Evaluate how strongly you feel about the topic you have chosen, whether you know the subject area well enough to write about it, and whether the topic is worth writing about at all (if this evaluation yields a poor result, choose another topic).

5. Survey a list of professional journals in your field and compare what each has to offer. Identify two or three journals in which you would like to have an article published. Set a realistic timeframe for submitting articles to these journals for review and publication.

6. Find a mentor who is willing to support you in achieving your publishing goals.

3 | THE WRITING PROCESS

'the work is always accomplished one word at a time.'
—King (2000, p. 122)

'I try to write down every word with caution and a sense of craft, as though I were carving hieroglyphics on the tomb of a well-loved king. Writing is both hard labor and one of the most pleasant forms that fanaticism can take. I take infinite care in how a sentence sounds to me.'
—Conroy (1998, p. 57)

The process of writing begins the moment you decide to write *and* physically sit down to commence the work. The challenge, once you start writing, is not merely to keep focused on what you are doing and to keep writing until the work has been completed, but to write *well*.

Most books addressing the art, craft and science of successful writing acknowledge that an essential ingredient of 'good' writing is *style*. As the veteran writer Majorie Holmes (1969, p. 107) points out in her classic text *Writing the Creative Article*:

Style is important. Of style, Aristotle said, 'it is not enough to know what to say; we must also say it in the right way.' The first impression an editor gets from any piece of writing is the author's style. The subject may be a good one, the words sufficient—like clothes, they may *cover* it; but if they are sloppy, prosaic or dull, or merely inappropriate, the editor has to drive himself [sic] to get through the manuscript.

The question is: what is style, and can it be taught?

THE ELEMENTS OF STYLE

At its most basic, style is '*your* way of writing'—the expression of your personality as an author (Holmes 1969, p. 108). A more substantive definition of style is:

> The art of clear, effective, and readable writing. The rhythm that makes a sentence sound right to the mental ear. The ruthless cutting out of phrases that only clutter and impede this special music. And always, always, the patient, painstaking search for the perfect combination of words and phrases that will create this mental music and express what is to be said in the most moving and effective way. (Holmes 1969, p. 107)

Writing with 'voice'

Style can also be defined as writing that expresses or carries the author's 'voice', without which the writing might be 'dead'. Peter Elbow's (1998, pp. 287–8) views on this issue are worth quoting at length. He writes:

> Writing with no voice is dead, mechanical, faceless. It lacks any sound. Writing with no voice *may* be

saying something true, important, or new; it may be logically organized; it may even be a work of genius. But it is as though the words came through some kind of mixer rather than uttered by a person. Extreme lack of voice is characteristic of bureaucratic memos, technical engineering writing, much sociology, many textbooks . . . Nobody is home here. In its extreme form, no voice is the army-manual of style. But the sad truth is that the careful writing of most people lacks voice . . .

Voice, in contrast, is what most people have in their speech but lack in their writing—namely, a sound or texture—the sound of 'them'. We recognize most of our friends on the phone before they say who they are. A few people get their voice into their writing. When you read a letter or something else they've written, it has the sound of them. It feels as though writing with voice has life in it.

Sometimes a writer's style may be so strong that others can recognise it without knowing the identity of the author. For example, a publisher informed me recently: 'Your manuscript reviewed very well. You might also like to know that one of the reviewers responded, "I don't know who wrote this chapter, but I bet it was Megan-Jane Johnstone—it *sounds* like her".'

Can style be taught?
Many ask whether style can be taught. The short answer to this question is: yes, no, maybe. In at least one fundamental sense, style is elusive in much the same way

that 'rhythm or good taste or passion' is elusive, and hence not something that can be taught (Holmes 1969, p. 107). In another sense, style can be 'taught' in that writers can be shown how to *develop* and *improve* their style. According to Holmes (1969, p. 108), there are two cardinal rules for improving and developing style:

- by writing—not just occasionally, but regularly
- by developing an awareness of the style of others—notably by reading and studying the work of others.

On this latter point, William Zinsser (1998, p. 35) advises:

Make a habit of reading what is written today and what has been written by earlier masters. Writing is learned by imitation. If anyone asked me how I learned to write, I'd say I learned by reading men and women who were doing the kind of writing *I* wanted to do and trying to figure out how they did it. But cultivate the best models.

Holmes advocates the following specific strategies for developing your own writing style:

- expose yourself to the kinds of things you want to write about
- read widely (not just one author)
- mark passages that please you and reread them, noting why they please you
- underscore the good figures of speech, count their frequency and taste their flavour

- read the works just before you sit down to write (adapted from Holmes 1969, pp. 109–10).

THE PRINCIPLES OF STYLE

The development of a good writing style—like the development of good conduct—can be guided by a set of principles. Some such principles, or 'secrets of style' as Marjorie Holmes refers to them, are:

1. aim for simplicity
2. avoid trite phrases and clichés
3. use figures of speech appropriately
4. avoid euphemisms, slang and colloquialisms
5. choose your words carefully (seek the 'right' word; avoid rare and difficult words)
6. avoid repeating key words (unless for emphasis or effect)
7. avoid redundancy
8. use alliteration
9. keep sentences as short as possible
10. develop a feel for rhythm
11. be original (adapted from Holmes 1969, pp. 110–22; *Style Manual* 1994; Manser and Curtis 2002).

Aim for simplicity

The key to good writing is *simplicity*—that is, saying what you mean in a clear, direct and simple (though engaging) manner. To achieve simplicity in your work, follow these steps:

1. write the work
2. take a 'cooling off' period

3. return to the work after a few days (or, if time is of the essence, at the very least after a night's sleep)
4. reread it
5. search for anything that detracts from what you mean to say or obscures its clarity
6. remove any words, views, or expressions that are superfluous (Holmes 1969; Zinsser 1998).

Many writers think that using 'big words' (for example, 'accede to' versus 'allow'; 'acquiesce' versus 'agree'; 'reside' versus 'live') and discipline-exclusive jargon enhances the merits and profundity of what they are writing (for a comparative list of common *complex* versus *simple* words, see Manser and Curtis 2002, pp. 205–7). In reality, however, jargon and big words often obscure what the writer is trying to say and may make their work largely inaccessible and meaningless to others. Sometimes, of course, it is genuinely difficult to avoid discipline-specific jargon. For instance, in my writing on ethics and bioethics, words like 'ethics', 'morality', 'rights', 'duties', 'deontology', 'teleology', and so forth, are often critical to the discussion I am advancing and, on account of having specific philosophic meanings, not able to be avoided. To overcome the problem of these words possibly making my writing obscure and unclear—especially when writing for a novice audience—I explain upfront what these terms mean.

The hallmark of a 'good' writer is someone who can make complex ideas accessible and meaningful. Furthermore, as Holmes (1969, p. 111) correctly argues, 'A good mind with a good idea should strive to make that idea understood'. Obscurity, suggests Holmes, is *not* the mark of profundity and should be avoided at all costs.

One strategy that can be used to keep a check on the use of words whose meanings may be obscure to others is to:

- identify the 'big words' in your work
- ask yourself whether the inclusion of these word is really necessary, or whether there are other simpler words that could be used (to assist in the search for simpler words, consult a dictionary and/or a thesaurus)
- seek the advice of an 'ally reader' on whether the sections of writing you are concerned about are as obscure as you think (beware also of being overly self-critical).

Avoid trite phrases and clichés

Clichés in writing are regarded as being the 'kiss of death' to a manuscript—not least because they undermine the process of continuing originality that is so critical to achieving stylish writing (Holmes 1969, p. 112; Zinsser 1998, p. 237). According to William Zinsser (1998, p. 237) if you want to give your readers a taste of something fresh, use words and expressions that have 'surprise, strength and precision'. Words that don't have these qualities should not be used. The following are some examples of clichés:

- 'At the cutting edge'
- 'The bottom line is . . .'
- 'While there's life there's hope'
- 'When push comes to shove . . .'

- 'It was too good to be true'
- 'To explore every avenue'
- 'The powers that be'
- 'You don't have to be a rocket scientist to figure it out . . .'
- 'Few and far between'.

It is generally accepted by those writing about writing that clichés should be avoided unless you are an extremely experienced writer with the capacity to use a cliché in a deliberate, clever and surprising way to emphasis a point. One way of achieving this is by treating the phrase 'contrapuntally'—that is, by turning it about. The technique of 'contrapuntal turnabout' is discussed later in this chapter.

Use figures of speech appropriately

A *figure of speech* is 'an expression of language, such as a simile, metaphor, or personification, by which the usual or literal meaning of the word is not employed'; figures of speech are used to add 'rhetorical force or interest to a spoken or written passage' (*Collins English Dictionary* 1995; *The New Oxford Dictionary of English* 2001).

The decision to use figures of speech in written work needs to be considered carefully. Like clichés, if they are not used skilfully, they can be a kiss of death to a manuscript. *Mixing* figures of speech can be especially problematic since this can confuse both the image and associated point that the writer is trying to make. On this latter point, Holmes cautions, 'Better no images at all than mixed ones' (1969, p. 115).

Having said this, using figures of speech skilfully can be a very useful device to:

- emphasise a point
- add life and colour to your style
- generally enhance the coherency and integrity of your work.

A good example of how a figure of speech can be used successfully to emphasise a point—and to do so succinctly and with power—can be found by looking at Dr Bob Brown, a leading figure in the Australian conservation movement. One of Dr Brown's great talents is his ability to use metaphors effectively and to create pictures with words in order to both explain and emphasise a point. One example of this is his reported comment that, 'Flooding the Franklin [a wilderness area situated in the State of Tasmania] would be like putting a scratch across the Mona Lisa or across a Beethoven record'.

Commenting on Bob Brown's capacity to use picturesque speech, Jonathan West writes:

> When someone says 'we're just putting a little road through a wilderness area,' he [Bob Brown] is able to create a picture by saying 'that's like putting a scratch across the face of the Mona Lisa. The vast majority of the Mona Lisa is intact but the scratch spoils it.' The long, detailed, technical explanation about the way in which the road would reduce the amount of wilderness square kilometres would have nothing like

the same impact as a simple word image like that (West, quoted in Thompson 2000, pp. 51–2).

Avoid euphemisms, slang and colloquialisms

A euphemism is an inoffensive word or phrase that is substituted for a word or phase that may be considered offensive or hurtful. Examples include: 'passed away' (instead of died), 'ethnic cleansing' (instead of genocide), 'passed wind' (instead of farted). Since the use of euphemisms can be misleading, the consensus is they are best avoided (*Style Manual* 1994, 1.31).

Slang refers to vocabulary (characteristically metaphorical in nature) that falls outside of the standard form of language; a colloquialism is similar to slang in that it refers to an informal expression that is appropriate only in certain contexts and conversations. Examples include:

- 'Buckley's chance' (Australian and New Zealand slang for 'no chance at all')
- 'cocky' (Australian informal for 'cockatoo', a native bird, or New Zealand and Australian slang for 'a cow farmer'; also US and Canadian slang for 'someone who is overly sure of themselves')
- 'dilly' (US and Canadian slang for 'a person or thing that is remarkable'; in Australia and New Zealand it slang for quite the opposite and refers to 'someone who is remarkably silly')
- 'wally' (general slang for 'stupid person').

Slang and colloquialisms can be misunderstood, confuse readers and can generally undermine the quality of formal writing, and for these reasons are best avoided.

Choose your words carefully

Good writing is both an art and craft. It fundamentally involves the art of carefully crafting words into expressions that have the capacity to convey images and ideas with strength, precision and originality. Good writing makes an impression on the minds of its readers; depending on the subject matter, good writing also has the capacity to change lives.

A critical ingredient of good writing is the careful selection of words. No effort should be spared in searching for and selecting the 'right' word.

As already mentioned, the use of 'big words' and rare or difficult words is not good writing; moreover the use of such words is likely to confound readers and to cause them to feel frustrated and irritated. A frustrated reader is not a good outcome; among other things it can lead to a 'lost reader' and ultimately a lost audience.

Choosing the right word means you need to know the correct meanings of the words you are using. This may seem obvious, nevertheless, it is surprising how often writers overlook this crucial point. Often we think we know the meaning of a given word, only to discover at some later point (either in conversation with others or when consulting a dictionary) that it may in fact have quite a different meaning to what we thought.

It is important to be mindful that language is not static and that the meaning of words can and do change over time. Overwhelming evidence of this can be found in the twenty-volume *Oxford English Dictionary* where discussion on the definition of a word, its origins and different meanings can run into *pages*, not merely paragraphs.

Since words are the essential ingredients of writing, it is essential that all writers get into the habit of using dictionaries. I would add that all writers should also get into the habit of using *different* dictionaries. For example, in *Bioethics: A nursing perspective*, when discussing possible meanings of the word 'dignity', I cite definitions from three leading dictionaries—the *Collins English Dictionary*, the *Oxford English Dictionary* and *Webster's Dictionary* (Johnstone 1999a, p. 241). My reason for doing this was simple: each of these dictionaries offered a slightly different perspective on the meaning of the word 'dignity' that was both thought provoking and added substance to the discussion being advanced.

Using the wrong words—or using words that are inappropriate—may prove to be not only embarrassing for a writer but, more seriously, may undermine the meaning, purpose, significance and integrity of a writer's work. One way to avoid this situation is to care deeply about your writing and about the words that you ultimately choose to use. On this point, Holmes (1969, p. 119) advises:

> The truly creative writer cares deeply about words— enough to take infinite pains to make his [or her] writing style as nearly perfect as possible. This means a constant quest to find the one word that most precisely expresses his [or her] thought . . . Good

writing can only come from this quality of deep caring, and this willingness to work toward perfection. Bad writing comes sometimes less from lack of talent than from sheer carelessness.

Avoid repeating key words

It is easy, when writing, to fall into the trap of repeating key words. All writers do it, most unintentionally, some even carelessly, but either way, rarely are they used with good effect. Unless there is an intended purpose behind repeating key words, such as to emphasise or underscore a crucial point, this practice is best avoided. Holmes (1969, p. 118) crafted the following paragraph as an example of tardy repetitious writing:

> I cannot tell you how moved I am to come here and try to dedicate this ground. As I move toward this ground and tried to think how to dedicate it I realised that I had dedicated myself to a task which cannot be done. This ground was already dedicated, I thought, by the death of the men who died.

Although it is best to avoid repeating key words, this does not mean that there is no place for utilising the technique of 'repetition' as a creative device in writing.

Some writers are able to skilfully use the technique of repeating key words with good effect. A famous example of this can be found in Martin Luther King's legendary 'I have a dream' speech, delivered on the steps at the Lincoln Memorial in Washington DC on 28 August 1963 (this speech can be downloaded from the Martin

Luther King website at <http://web66.coled.umn.edu/ new/MLK/MLK.html>) in which Dr King repeated the words 'I have a dream' eight times, and the words 'Let freedom ring' seven times in his concluding comments.

There are other poignant repetitions in King's speech, which work to great effect. For instance, when referring to the level of dissatisfaction among Black Americans concerning their lack of civil rights, King (1963) wrote:

> *We can never be satisfied* as long as our bodies, heavy with the fatigue of travel, cannot gain lodging in the motels of the highways and the hotels of the cities. *We cannot be satisfied* as long as the Negro's basic mobility is from a smaller ghetto to a larger one. *We can never be satisfied* as long as a Negro in Mississippi cannot vote and a Negro in New York believes he has nothing for which to vote. No, no, *we are not satisfied*, and *we will not be satisfied* until justice rolls down like waters and righteousness like a mighty stream. [emphasis added]

In anticipation of Black Americans eventually succeeding in achieving the civil rights and freedom they sought, and how this would be heralded, King concluded his speech by quoting the words from an old Negro spiritual, ' "Free at last! Free at last! Thank God Almighty, we are free at last!" ' (Incidentally, King's speech is also full of rich examples of the effective use of figures of speech; one example is, 'Let us not seek to satisfy our thirst for freedom by drinking from the cup of bitterness and hatred'.)

The words used in King's speech demonstrate that

repetitions can be used intentionally, powerfully and with good effect. The key is to be *careful* in the way you use these. As Holmes (1969, p. 122) points out, it is the 'careless, unnecessary repetitions that clutter your style and that editors deplore'.

In order to avoid careless repetitions in your work:

- take care in the original crafting of the work
- take a 'cooling off' period
- reread the work (or have a mentor or friendly critic read the work) and search actively for any repetitions
- remove repeated words that serve no purpose and/or have no effect in terms of emphasising a point.

Avoid redundancy

In language, words or expressions are generally considered to be redundant when they are *tautological*, that is, they 'merely repeat elements of the meaning already conveyed' (*Collins English Dictionary* 1995). Expressions can also be redundant when they are verbose, that is, when they contain an excess of words that focus on insignificant detail.

Some notable examples of redundancy include:

- *yellow jaundice*
- *sugar diabetes*
- *two twins*
- 'will the funds available be *adequate enough*' (versus, 'will the funds available be adequate')
- 'the older residents could now climb the stairs *safely and not get hurt*' (versus 'the older residents could now climb the stairs safely')

- '*apparently* the Chief Executive resigned *ostensibly* for health reasons' (versus, 'apparently the Chief Executive resigned for health reasons' or 'the Chief Executive resigned ostensibly for health reasons').

Tips for avoiding redundancy in your work, include:

- when writing, do not labour a point unnecessarily
- take a 'cooling off' period
- reread the work for redundancies
- remove any redundancies.

Use alliteration

Alliteration, defined as 'the occurrence of the same letter or sound at the beginning of adjacent or closely connected words' (*New Oxford English Dictionary* 2001), is another technique that can be used to add life, rhythm and uniqueness to a writer's style. More commonly associated with poetry and tongue twisters (for example, 'Peter Piper picked a peck of pickled pepper') many writers overlook this device as a stylish writing technique. Like other creative writing techniques, however, it needs to be applied with craft and skill if it is to work effectively.

Alliteration can be used powerfully and effectively in titles of works, in an opening or a concluding paragraph, and in the general body of a work. For example:

Titles:
- 'Pumped Philippoussis tames a tough Thai' (headline in *The Age*, 16 January 2003, p. 1)
- *Health, Hope and Healing* (Tate 1989)

- *Lewd Women and Wicked Witches* (Hester 1992)
- *Situating the Self* (Benhabib 1992)
- *Professions and Patriarchy* (Witz 1992)
- *On Lies, Secrets, and Silence—selected prose 1966–1978* (Rich 1979)
- *Cruel Compassion: Psychiatric control of society's unwanted* (Szasz 1994).

Opening paragraph: 'Five score years ago, a great American, in whose symbolic shadow we stand signed the Emancipation Proclamation' (Martin Luther King, 1963, opening sentence to his 'I have a dream' speech). Note how the 's' sounds add smoothness and rhythm to his opening statement.

General body: 'Just as a stopped clock can bear permanent witness to the exact time of a particular atrocity, so the memory of a particular event in our past can have the power to close off the future and stop our life' (Holloway 2002, p. 32).

Keep sentences as short as possible

Another critical feature of a good writing style is *readability*. Readability of a work can be enhanced greatly by keeping sentences short and to the point. Some sentences will, of course, need to be longer than others depending on what is being expressed. Nevertheless, there is *always* room for improvement.

When I first started writing as a university undergraduate student in the early 1980s I wrote long, convoluted sentences. Aware that I had a problem (one day I barely passed an assignment when I had expected to get an 'A' pass), I approached a very patient study-skills teacher for assistance. On my first visit, the teacher gently pointed out to me that one of the sentences in this assignment (I had given it to her for feedback) contained over 60 words and that several other sentences contained only slightly less words than that. I learned a valuable lesson that day:

- all sentences in a work need to be examined carefully
- long sentences can always be improved, either by being 'broken' into smaller sentences or by having unnecessary words and phrases deleted
- never underestimate the value of a mentor or friendly reader who is willing to critique your work and who can be trusted to pick you up on your blind spot when it comes to writing long sentences.

Develop a feel for rhythm

Rhythm, the periodic or regular recurrence of sound or movement, is perhaps more commonly associated with music than with writing. Yet rhythm is just as important to good writing as it to good music. Furthermore, as William Zinsser (1998, p. 37) advises, 'considerations of sound and rhythm should be woven through everything you write'.

The best way to get a sense of the rhythm (or lack of rhythm) in your own writing is to read it aloud to yourself. By reading your work aloud you can 'both hear and feel' its rhythm through speech.

Zinsser (1998, p. 37) states that he writes 'entirely by ear and read[s] everything aloud before letting [his work] go out into the world'. I also read my writing aloud to myself. I listen for its rhythm, and note where it is lacking. When reading aloud, I note where there exists a clutter of words, and where there is a need for pause and punctuation. Over the years, many students have told me that I 'speak like I write'. The reality is, that I write like I speak. Sometimes I literally dictate aloud to myself what I am writing.

There are many ways to cultivate rhythm in your writing. One way is to study the rhythm in the writing of others. A good place to start would be to read the speeches written by Martin Luther King (see Martin Luther King website address earlier in this chapter). Other useful resources include:

- William Safire's (1997) *Lend Me Your Ears: Great speeches in history* (which includes speeches and works by many notable figures in history, including the ancient Greek philosophers Pericles and Socrates, the Roman emperor Julius Ceaser, the former English prime minister Sir Winston Churchill, the former US president John F. Kennedy, and many others)
- Peter Thompson's (2000) *The Secrets of the Great Communicators* (a book and CD package that includes a CD recording of the four-part series of the same title originally broadcast on ABC radio in Australia).

Be original

Originality—the ability to create something fresh, new and unusual—is another important ingredient of style. And, like style, it rests just as much on skill, focus and hard work as it does on talent, intuition and creative imagination. While the work of some writers is clearly more original than the work of others, there are nevertheless ways in which originality in style can be enhanced and improved. For example, you can draw on the techniques of:

- 'lateral thinking' and 'thinking outside the square' advocated by the tactician and provocateur Edward de Bono (for a succinct summary of de Bono's many works, see Dudgeon 2001)
- creative and critical thinking advocated by the Vincent Ruggiero (1995), a pioneer and author in the field of critical and creative thinking.

Using the contrapuntal device (see below) can also enhance originality as can using the various other style techniques already discussed in this chapter. Being passionately and almost fanatically interested in what you are writing is another means of enhancing originality. As Zinsser (1998, p. 247) concludes:

> Living is the trick. Writers who write interestingly tend to be men and women who keep themselves interested. That's almost the whole point of becoming a writer.

THE CONTRAPUNTAL DEVICE

A little-known technique for enhancing writing style is the contrapuntal device—a counterpoint technique whereby a phrase, such as a cliché or figure of speech, is 'turned about'. This technique, also referred to tautologically as the *contrapuntal turnabout*, can give a work what William Safire (1997, p. 19) calls 'quotable nuggets'.

There are many famous examples of contrapuntal expressions. For example, Abraham Lincoln used the device to switch 'the cynical "might is right" to the moral "right makes might"' (Safire 1997, p. 19). Similarly, John F. Kennedy used the device to switch the pessimistic 'never negotiate out of fear' to the optimistic 'never fearing to negotiate' (Safire 1997, p. 19). Other examples are:

- 'We cannot live within the past, but the past lives within us' (the late Charlie Perkins, Aboriginal leader and activist, dedication and postscript to the film *One Night the Moon* directed by Rachel Perkins, his daughter and a noted Australian filmmaker)
- 'What is the point? To destroy a man who seeks the truth or to destroy the truth so that no man can seek it?' (*The X-Files*, 'The Truth', 2003)
- 'The second, and more reliable, method [for achieving inner contentment] is not to have what we want but rather to want and appreciate what we have' (His Holiness the Dalai Lama and Cutler 1998, p. 29)
- 'The pessimist sees the difficulties in every opportunity. The optimist, the opportunity in every difficulty' (Jacks 2002, p. 63).

DRAFTING AND REDRAFTING

A key part of writing is the process of *drafting* and *redrafting* the work. All writing initially is a draft—a *preliminary* work—since rarely, if at all, is a work word perfect from the

outset and almost always will require at least some amendment. Some works, of course, will require more or less
drafting and redrafting than others, depending on the
nature of the work and experience of the author. But,
ultimately, no writing process is complete until the
drafting–redrafting process is complete.

Many writers (especially novice writers) baulk at the
prospect and experience of having to redraft their work
(students writing theses get particularly discouraged by
this process). Some writers, however, rightly embrace the
redrafting phase as a kind of 'quality control' of their
writing (Dunn 1999, p. 89) and as an opportunity to
craft an exemplary piece of work—an attitude that often
brings rich rewards. For example, the Russian novelist,
short story writer and philosopher, Leo Tolstoy (1828–
1910), author of the two monumental novels *War and
Peace* and *Anna Karenina*, is reputed to have gone
through and rewritten his first novel *War and Peace* eight
times, and was still making corrections on the final galley
proofs of the work (Carver, in Fishman 2000, p. 139).
Both of these works became classics and remain in print.

Redrafting a work is just as critical as the original
drafting of the work. Your work's success may ultimately
depend on this process, provided it is done well. One
reason for this is that it enables you to check that the
principles of style have been upheld and to make amendments if they have not been. Redrafting provides you
with an opportunity to check that:

- the work has been written in a clear, direct and simple
  manner

- trite phrases and clichés have been avoided
- figures of speech have been used appropriately
- the right words have been chosen, and rare and difficult words avoided
- repetitions have been avoided or, if used, handled in a skilful and effective manner
- redundancies have been avoided
- alliteration has been used appropriately
- sentences are of an appropriate length, and are shortened if too long
- the work is read aloud and checked for rhythm
- the final work demonstrates the hallmarks of originality
- the work has come together as a coherent, accessible and meaningful whole.

SUMMARY

To produce 'good writing' it is essential to apply the elements and principles of style. The key element of style is writing with personality and voice. Through regular practice, mentoring and exposure to the unique styles of other writers, a writing style can be developed and improved. A good writing style, in turn, can be developed and improved by upholding the principles of style that have as their ultimate purpose the production of writing that is readable, meaningful, original, memorable and successful. These principles also underscore the point that it is only by sitting down and writing and, at the appropriate time, rewriting a work that the job of writing gets done.

EXERCISES

1. Make a list of authors whose writing styles you admire.

2. Study these authors' works and note the 'secrets' of their style.

3. Examine your own work (for example, an essay written for a university course, a journal article you may have had published) and note the extent to which you have upheld (or not upheld) the principles of style and where improvements could be made.

4 | THE WINNING HABITS OF SUCCESSFUL AUTHORS

'You must once and for all give up being worried about success and failures. Don't let that concern you. It's your duty to go on working steadily day by day, quite steadily, to be prepared for mistakes, which are inevitable, and for failures.'
—Anton Chekhov, quoted in Fishman (2000, p. 123)

'Success doesn't happen overnight. A positive attitude, a professional approach and perseverance are usually behind "sudden" success.'
—Day (1993, p. 8)

Before settling down to the business of producing a written work suitable for publication, there remains here one more task to complete: notably, to examine the winning habits of successful authors. Since habits, by their nature, are hard to break—especially bad habits—it is important that, as a new writer, you focus on cultivating good writing habits right from the start.

THE WILL TO WRITE
To succeed as a writer you must not only *want* to write but have *the will to write*. The will to write is taken here to mean 'not just a desire to write, or an impulse to write, but an

overpowering determination to write' [emphasis added] (McAlpine 2000a, p. 9). To put this another way, if you are really serious about writing you must have a *passion to write*—almost to the point of being fanatical. As Ray Bradbury (1992, p. 4) points out in *Zen in the Art of Writing*:

> . . . if you are writing without zest, without gusto, without love, without fun, you are only half a writer . . . you are not being yourself. You don't even know yourself. For the first thing a writer should be is—excited.

Passion for writing—like any calling—must, however, also be matched by fortitude. Gregg Levoy (1997, p. 74) explains that having a calling is:

> like entering into a committed relationship. If you're going to promise to be with someone, you'd better be in love or share a common purpose, because you know that being in a relationship is a difficult struggle. There has to be some higher purpose for it, otherwise you won't be able to maintain it.

The will to write is also much more than the will to be a *writer*.

I cannot imagine anything more deadly to a person's aspiration to be a writer than a lack of will, a lack of commitment, apathy, a passionate desire to *avoid* the task. If you do not have a passionate desire—the will—to write, and you lack commitment to engaging in the process of writing, then your aspirations should perhaps be focused elsewhere.

WRITE ABOUT WHAT YOU KNOW

It is much easier to write about what you know than what you don't know. One reason for this is that in the realm of the known lie many seeds of thought and ideas. If you know a subject area well, you will be in a much better position to generate critical questions and to advance critical discussion on that subject. Equally important, by writing about what you know you will be in a better position to anticipate the length of time you will need to write a work and, crucially, to meet publication timelines.

Writing about what you know also has the paradoxical effect of helping you to get known for/by what you write. In my case, I have written extensively on the subject of bioethics since the late 1980s. Bioethics is the field in which I have trained academically, have developed in-depth knowledge and have specialised. Ironically, I am known more for the books that I have produced, than for my knowledge of the subject matter per se. Nurses have often greeted me with 'Oh, you are the nurse who writes books', even though they have not read them and know little about my work as an ethicist.

WRITE ABOUT WHAT INTERESTS YOU

The importance of writing about what interests you can never be overemphasised. On the rare occasions that I have agreed to write something about which I have had little interest, I have, as they say, come horribly unstuck. In one notable instance several years ago, I had a contract with a major international publishing house to write a chapter for a book being edited by two highly reputable international authors. Shortly before the due submission date I had to withdraw my contribution because, quite simply, it was badly written and I just could not find the will or the insights necessary to rewrite and improve the draft to comply with what the academic editors wanted. On reflection I realised that I should never have agreed to write the chapter in the first place. My decision to participate in the publishing program was for the wrong reasons, notably, to have the opportunity to work with two high-profile international authors, rather than to communicate ideas on an issue about which I felt strongly.

If you do not write about what interests you and what you find deeply significant and meaningful it will be difficult to progress, to develop as a writer, and to write meaningfully and in a way that will touch your audience. It will also be difficult to find the motivation and fort- itude necessary to go the distance, to travel that long and sometimes tortuous path to success. In short, if you do not write about what you are interested in, it will be difficult for you to develop a writing career.

KEEP A NOTEBOOK

It is always important to be open to and keep track of new ideas and thoughts pertinent to your writing. New ideas and thoughts can often come at the most unex- pected (and inconvenient) times such as when you are having a shower, driving a car, reading a book, watching a movie, having a conversation with a friend or colleague, overhearing someone else's conversation or when you are about to go off to sleep at night. It is important that these ideas and thoughts are noted down as soon as possible otherwise you risk losing them.

It is good practice to have a designated notebook (and a special pen) for writing down ideas and thoughts pertinent to your writing. This notebook should be distinctive or of a favourite colour, have a high-quality texture and carry the title 'Writing notebook' or something similar to reflect its special purpose. In addition, it is useful (and also good practice) to have a number of smaller-sized notebooks that can be accessed easily, such as from your pocket, a handbag or briefcase, or the glove box of your car. Keeping 'work in progress' notes is also a good way of keeping a record of the development of your thoughts and will enable you to assess your development as a writer. Having a special pen adds to the art and process of writing. My special pen is a gold fountain pen.

PRACTICE WRITING

Like all skills, writing must be practised if competence (if not excellence) is to be achieved and sustained. Just as professional tennis players and professional musicians must practice for long hours to perfect their skill, so too must writers. On this point, Ray Bradbury (1990, p. xiii) reminds us:

> Remember that pianist who said that if he did not practice every day *he* would know, if he did not practice for two days, the *critics* would know, after three days, his *audiences* would know . . . A variation of this is true for writers.

There are many opportunities (both formal and informal) for practising writing during the course of a day. As stated in the opening chapter to this book, most clinicians in health care spend some time writing as part of their day-to-day professional duties. Some may spend as much as 20 per cent of their working day writing. Whether writing a short email message, case notes on a patient, or writing a larger work such as a report on a quality assurance matter, these are all wonderful opportunities for practising the art, craft and science of writing. Furthermore it is important to remember that 'Any writing helps you with any other writing' (McAlpine 2000a, p. 11).

One of the great things for me personally about being employed as an academic is that hardly a day goes by without writing of some kind or another being required of me. I therefore get to practice writing almost everyday. I value this opportunity deeply and try always to take great care in what I write, even with the smallest piece. I will, for example, pay as much attention to crafting the words of an email as I do when crafting the words of a more major work. I do not always achieve a word-perfect message, but the practice is going on nonetheless and I always feel the benefit of that practice. As well as enabling me to constantly refine my writing skills, my daily writing at work keeps me primed so that if and when I need to sit down to write a larger work my mind and soul is ready in an instant to proceed.

Learning to write takes practice and practice takes time. The trick is to be 'realistic and patient with ourselves while we are learning' (DeSalvo 1999, p. 33).

MAKE TIME

One of the biggest complaints by aspiring writers (especially those who are also busy professionals) is that they 'do not have time to write' or, if they do have some time, they are simply too exhausted at the end of the day to focus on the job of writing. There is only one solution to this problem: *make time*. If you are serious about writing you have to find some way of:

- cultivating and preserving your energy for writing
- taking time out of your busy schedule to write.

Making time for writing and taking 'time out' to write requires *discipline*. The amount of time you need and how regularly you need to schedule your writing time will depend on a number of things, including:

- the nature of the work
- the schedule for completion of the work
- the conditions under which you work best; for example, some people work better under pressure and tend to work more efficiently the less time they have— the more time they have, the more time they waste; in contrast, others need more time and less pressure in order to work productively (Rankin 2001, pp. 79–80).

Depending on your writing goals, you may only need to set aside a few hours every day (for example, two to four hours), or one or two days per week to write. In some instances (for example, when undertaking a major work) you may need to take time off work for several weeks and possibly even months in order to write. While there is no 'one size fits all' program for time management, one thing is sure: *you need to set up a writing schedule and commit yourself to it.* A writing schedule must include:

- the identification of specific writing projects
- the number of words required per project
- timelines.

Once you have prepared your writing schedule place it in a prominent place, such as above your writing desk, so that it is kept before you. (An example of a writing schedule is included as Figure 4.1 in this chapter). Once you have done this, using either a standard year planner or a Gannt chart (see Figure 4.2 in this chapter), block out or mark with a highlighter or arrows the days each week that you plan to work on your projects and the specific tasks that you have chosen. For example, when preparing the manuscript for this book, I worked strictly to a day planner on which I had marked the dates (representing self-prescribed timelines) by which I had to complete each chapter. While working to this schedule, I started writing at 9 a.m. each morning and did not stop writing until I had completed all the tasks I had set myself for that day. Sometimes the task took me just eight hours of writing time to complete; other times it took me between twelve and sixteen hours writing time to complete (for instance, I would start writing at 8 a.m. and would not stop until midnight). On the occasions when a particular section or chapter was evidently going to take longer than I had anticipated, I would revise the writing timeline accordingly, although still within a strict schedule. As I completed each task, I marked it off with a tick to give me encouragement. By following this regime, I completed the first draft of the manuscript for this book in just fourteen days.

Figure 4.1: Example of a writing schedule

Project	Word Limit	Timeline
1. Journal article: 'Poor working conditions and the capacity of nurses to provide moral care'	4000 words	Submit for review: June 2002 Journal: *Contemporary Nurse*
2. Book manuscript: *Effective Writing for Health Professionals*	50 000 words	Submit to Allen & Unwin: February 2003
3. Book manuscript: *Bioethics, 4th edn*	408 pages	Submit to Elsevier Science: November 2003

Facing the task of writing a work of 4000 words in length or 40 000 words in length may seem overwhelming in contexts where time is paramount. One way of putting the task into perspective is to remind yourself that there are 365 days in a year. Once you have completed all the preparatory work for your writing (that is, have searched out all your references and other material relevant to the project), if you can manage to write even 400 words a day you face the very real prospect of being able to complete a draft of a journal article in ten days and a small book (like this one) in 40 days. Even if you were to write only 200 words a day, it would be possible, by these calculations, to write *several* journal articles each year, not just one.

Beware, however, of setting your daily writing schedule too low. Stephen King (2000, p. 121) argues that beginning professional writers should write *at least* 1000 words a day, six days per week; anything less than this, he suggests, and 'you'll lose the urgency and immediacy of your story'.

While I would only suggest you adopt King's prescription if you are working as a full-time professional writer, his advice is pertinent even for causal writers: if you do not write a minimum amount of words each day or week, you risk losing the impetus to write. More seriously for part-time writers, if you stop your daily writing when you have reached your set word-limit for the day, rather than when you have exhausted your thoughts and writing on the subject matter at hand, you can seriously interrupt the continuity of your thoughts and disrupt the entire writing process. Such disruption can be just as frustrating as not writing at all since, often, when you resume the task of writing it feels like you are having to start from the beginning all over again.

One way of avoiding having to go back to your original starting point each time you sit down to write, is to *compartmentalise* your writing. For instance, when working on a scholarly article, assign yourself the task of writing a specific section on a specified day designated on your scheduled writing. On day one, for example, focus exclusively on writing the introduction, day two focus on discussing the first point of your article (your first subheading), on day three focus on discussing your second point (second subheading), and so on (see Figure 4.2: Example of a Gannt chart); on the scheduled writing days that you don't feel productive, focus on completing mundane tasks, such as formulating a table, typing up your reference list or reading some additional material and making notes.

Figure 4.2: Example of a Gannt chart

Writing task	Weeks Beginning							
	6/1	13/1	20/1	27/1	3/2	10/2	17/2	24/2
Introduction	→							
Subheading 1		→						
Subheading 2			→					
Subheading 3				→				
Subheading 4					→			
Conclusion						→		
Review/redraft							—————→	
Submit for publication								→

Eventually, like the pieces of an exquisitely crafted patchwork quilt, all the completed sections of your work can be placed together as a coherent whole, ready for rereading and editing as a completed manuscript.

Serious writing is like a job and should be seen as such. Once you start it, you must be willing to 'shut the door'. As King (2000, p. 121) advises:

> The closed door is your way of telling the world and yourself that you mean business; you have made a serious commitment to write and intend to walk the walk as well as talk the talk.

DEVELOP A 'GOOD' WRITING STYLE

To succeed as a writer it is imperative that you develop a good writing style. As stated previously, style refers to *your* way of writing and the expression of *your* personality and voice as an author. Since this topic has already been considered in the previous chapter, I need only say here that it is imperative that authors continually develop and improve their own writing style.

READ PROLIFICALLY AND ATTENTIVELY

Anybody who is serious about writing must READ. Reading is an essential preparatory stage of the writing process. It is critical for the purposes of gaining information, generating ideas and generally researching the background to your topic. It also serves the critical purpose of helping you develop your own personal writing style (see also Dunn 1999, p. 67).

It is no coincidence that most successful writers are also avid readers who read *with attention*. This is because, as Stephen King (2000, p. 114) explains, 'Reading is the creative center of a writer's life'. It enables writers to get a sense of style and to constantly refine (and redefine) their own work. He also cautions, 'If you don't have time to read, you don't have the time (or the tools) to write. Simple as that'.

When you finish a manuscript, set it aside. There inevitably (and thankfully!) comes a point at which you can do nothing further to a work and it is time to submit it to a journal or a commercial publisher (whichever is relevant) for review. When that point comes, it is also time to move on to the next project. Sit down and start writing the next article or book or whatever else it is that you have scheduled to write. In this way you will maintain your momentum as a writer.

BE AN EXCELLENT RESEARCHER

To undertake research is to conduct a systematic investigation to establish 'facts' or to collect information on a subject. As Ann Hoffmann (1999, p. 1) correctly points out:

> Every writer, unless he [or she] is creating a work of pure fantasy, has to do research. The nature and depth of the research will vary enormously, according to the subject of the work, the field of writing (factual article, novel, biography, history, thesis, children's story, etc.) and whether it is intended for the academic, popular or juvenile market.

A professional or an academic article or book will only be as good as the search and research that has been undertaken to inform it. When preparing to write a work, you need to search for, think about, and collate information in a manner that ultimately leaves you and your readers feeling that no rock has been left unturned. Furthermore, always collect more information than you need. There is a common saying in photography circles that a photographer may need to take one hundred pictures in order to take the perfect one. Literature searching and researching for an article or a book you are writing involves a similar process: you may need to locate one hundred articles in order to find the perfect one—what I call the 'academic gems' for quoting in one's writing. See 'Preparation' in Chapter 5 for more on this subject.

HAVE A GREAT FILING SYSTEM

An effective filing system is essential for keeping in order and storing the material you collect to inform and reference your writing. To this end, a filing cabinet is just as important as a writing desk and computer. How you arrange your filing system is a matter of personal preference and may depend on the nature of the topic or topics you are writing on and the volume of material you have collected. For example, you may wish to organise your material:

- alphabetically according to author surname
- thematically according to subject matter/topics (for example: 'euthanasia', 'hope', 'quality of life', 'withholding food and fluids', 'whistleblowing')

- into specific projects (with a separate filing system for each work that is organised in one of the ways described above. For example, for the work *Effective Writing for Health Professionals* material is filed in author alphabetical order: Arblaster, Archer, Arias, etc.)
- using a combination of the above.

HAVE A FABULOUS HOME LIBRARY

Every writer needs his or her own professional library. You also need to visit bookshops as frequently as you visit supermarkets to check out what is on the shelves and to make purchases as your interest and needs demand.

Not all good books are available in libraries and sometimes it is only by purchasing books that you maintain ready access to the thoughts and ideas that are contained within them. Further, when writing books, there is something inspiring about being surrounded by them.

The number of books you should have will depend on your interests, finances, home storage capacity and passion for books. The celebrated Brazilian author, Paulo Coelho (author of *The Alchemist, Veronika Decides to Die,* and numerous other titles) reveals that he keeps his library to a maximum of 400 books. His decision to keep such a small collection of books is more for practical than ideological reasons: he came home one day and found all the book shelves that once housed a much larger collection of books had collapsed onto the floor. He worried at the time that had someone been there they might have been killed (Arias 2001, p. 166). I know of people whose homes are walled with books. I have 1200 books in my home library simply because there is not space to shelve more.

In your home library, ensure you also have a good reference book section that includes the following range of books:

- at least one good dictionary (preferably more); choices include:
  - *The Macquarie Dictionary* (which reflects common Australian usage)
  - *Collins English Dictionary* (which reflects Australian, New Zealand, Scottish, Irish, Canadian, South African, East African, West African, Indian, Caribbean and British regional English)
  - *Oxford English Dictionary* (which reflects Standard English)
  - *Webster's Dictionary* (which reflects American-English)
- a good thesaurus
- a good book of quotations (for example, *The Times Book of Quotations*, 2000)
- a good writing style manual (for example, the *Style Manual,* 6th edition 2002; *The Penguin Writer's Manual* by M. Manser and S. Curtis, 2002)
- the latest edition of the *New Fontana Dictionary of Modern Thought* (published by HarperCollins, London)
- discipline-specific dictionaries (for example, a dictionary of philosophy, dictionary of sociology, dictionary of psychology, and so forth)

- a good local writers' marketplace guide (for example, Rhonda Whitton's *The Australian Writer's Marketplace: A complete guide to being published in Australia* and the *Writers' & Artists' Yearbook*, which contains information pertinent to publishing in the UK, Ireland, USA and Australia).

GET FEEDBACK FROM OTHERS

At some stage during the writing process writers develop what I shall call a 'blind spot'. On account of being so close to their own work, writers can lose the discrimination necessary for judging and deciding what is and what is not working in their writing. This can result in writers being either *overly critical* of or *overly satisfied* with their work or, more often, somewhere between the two.

It is at this point that feedback from others (for example: colleagues, prospective readers, students, other writers) can be very useful in terms of either:

- reassuring the writer that their work is interesting, informative, reads well and is near completion—or *is* complete and ready for submission, or
- advising the writer where improvements could be made, such as by expanding a point, strengthening an argument, better signposting an idea, refining a sentence, filling in a knowledge gap, including a key-reference that appears to have been overlooked, removing redundancies, picking up typographical errors and other errors that even the most accustomed eye can miss.

The key to getting helpful feedback from others is to find a mentor or 'ally reader' who is informed, critical and able to give you sound, reliable and constructive feedback. Those who will merely tell you how wonderful your writing is or, conversely and discouragingly, how terrible your writing is, should be avoided. It is also important that you have a *trusting relationship* with your mentor or ally reader(s). Trust is important because if you do not trust the people who are giving you feedback it may be difficult to not only accept their advice but to surrender your work to them for feedback at all.

All but one of my published works (a small book chapter) has been read by at least one ally reader before being submitted for publication. Without exception, my ally readers have picked up areas in my writing that needed improvement and I have never regretted accepting and acting on their feedback. I reciprocate their goodwill by functioning as an ally reader and mentor for them.

All writers need to get into the habit of utilising ally readers to critique their own work; they can also learn a lot and help other writers by serving as ally readers *themselves.*

BE A MENTOR AND COACH TO YOURSELF

Ally readers can provide valuable mentorship to a writer. Ultimately, however, as a writer there is no better mentor than *yourself.* On the issue of self-mentorship, Jack London, author of *The Call of the Wild* (1903) and described as 'an icon of literary success and one of the two or three most popular American writers in the world', wrote: 'in the main I am self-educated; *have had no mentor but myself*' [emphasis added](quoted in Walker and Reesman 1999, p. ix).

Self-mentorship (or self-coaching) basically involves assisting yourself to achieve your writing goals and develop your writing career. Others can give you support and feedback, and so forth. They cannot, however (and indeed, should not) plan your writing goals, write your work, adopt a lifestyle that enables you to write, submit your work for publication, accepts the rewards and punishments of your work. In several respects, self-mentorship is a necessary precondition to being mentored by others: a *writer must first be willing to help himself/herself before seeking and accepting the help of others*.

ACCEPT THE REWARDS AND PUNISHMENTS

Like any career, writing has its rewards and punishments. The key to success as a writer is to accept the rewards and punishments *as they come*. In the case of the punishments, it is vital that these are approached with tolerance and patience, and viewed as a valuable opportunity to learn and to develop as a writer and as a person.

Rewards

Undoubtedly one of the greatest rewards—if not *the* greatest reward—of writing is seeing the work published, and the deep sense of satisfaction you experience when you finally succeed in achieving your writing goal. There is no feeling quite like seeing your work in print. There are, of course, many other rewards:

- receiving positive feedback from reviewers and critics
- learning that your work has 'made a difference' to the lives of others
- having the work nominated for and/or win a literary award
- seeing your work referenced in the work of others and making a significant contribution of knowledge to the field
- receiving a job promotion based on your publication track record
- receiving remuneration (such as royalties)
- being offered other publishing opportunities based on your publication track record
- gaining an international reputation and receiving kudos
- receiving encouragement to keep going.

Punishments

Publishing is a very demanding and competitive activity. And just as its rewards can be rich, its punishment can be painful and demeaning. The punishments of publishing are not insurmountable, however, and in many respects are merely a part of the rites of passage to becoming a successful writer. Among the most punishing of experiences for writers are the processes of:

- submission
- rejection
- criticism
- redundancy
- politics of envy.

Submission

When a work is completed, the writer submits the work for publication, or, in other words, *makes a submission* to a chosen publisher. The act of 'submission' can be a very trying and humbling experience for writers. For many, it is tantamount to an act of 'surrender' and literally marks the first step toward 'judgement day' in regard to the merits of the work *and* the credibility of its author. As Gregg Levoy (1997, p. 84) notes, it is perhaps no coincidence that 'the word writers use to describe the act of sending their work out into the world is *submission*. It is indeed a kind of surrender'.

Once a manuscript has been submitted for review, you then have to wait patiently to learn whether the work has been accepted or rejected for publication. If there is a delay in the review process, this waiting period can be a challenging time for writers, particularly if they are under pressure to publish a minimum number of articles in any one calendar year, as is the case with academics. A lengthy delay in the review process can have serious implications for academics if it undermines their capacity to achieve their publishing-related performance indicators.

Rejection

The rejection of manuscripts is commonplace and is part of the everyday reality of writing and publishing. If you get a rejection from a publisher, the important thing is *not to take it personally*. Rejections are common even for experienced and successful authors, and may not necessarily be a reflection of the quality of the manuscript or the topicality or importance of the work. It may simply be that there is not a *profitable market* for the work or it does not 'fit' with a publisher's program (Dunn 1999, p. 14). For example in 1999 I received the following rejection letter from a publisher in response to a proposal I had submitted for a book on the ethics of reporting child abuse:

27 October, 1999

Dear Megan-Jane

Thank you for your manuscript proposal entitled 'Reporting child abuse: ethics, politics and the health professions'. While the manuscript is current and very interesting I am afraid it has a limited market within Australia and New Zealand. I will undertake some initial research and contact you with my findings. Please allow for 4–6 weeks for this procedure to be completed.

In addition, I spoke to . . . our Marketing Manager, who told me you had been in contact with her about the proposal. She has already contacted the publishing editors . . . in the United Kingdom regarding your proposal. Unfortunately they already have a 'Child Abuse' book and believe another text, in this already limited market, would be detrimental.

Please contact me if you have any queries.

Yours sincerely
Health Science Editor

I submitted the book proposal (with a completed manuscript) to three other publishing companies and got much the same response. The rejection of the manuscript remains a source of great disappointment to me. I regard the subject matter as important and the work as arguably one of my best to date. But the fact remains that four reputable academic publishing houses have made the same judgement (based on their own market research and experience) that there is *no profitable market for the work*. Unless I am prepared to self-publish the work (which I am not), I have to accept this rejection and the commercial wisdom underpinning it.

Writers have no control over their manuscripts being rejected. They do, however, have control over *how they respond* to the rejections they receive. There is no point getting angry about a rejection notice since it will not change the outcome. A constructive response is to accept the rejection and 'move on'. Depending on what, if any, feedback has been received, a writer has the options of:

- *accepting* a reviewer's recommendations for amendment, revising the work and resubmitting it to the same publisher for further review and possible publication
- *rejecting* a reviewer's recommendations for amendment and submitting the manuscript to a different publisher for review and possible publication.

Either way it is important to put manuscript rejections into perspective. Although receiving a rejection letter is always disappointing, it does not signal the end of your writing career. If you persevere, develop the habits of other successful writers, remain focused on improving your writing skills and style, and remain determined to achieve your writing goals, the chances are you will succeed in getting your work published.

Sometimes, when dealing with a rejection, it can be helpful to talk to or to read about others who have also been through such an experience. The following example of a rejection slip from a Chinese economics journal, quoted in the *Financial Times*, is worth quoting here since it provides a timely reminder to writers to keep the whole process of writing, publishing and rejection by editors in perspective:

> We have read your manuscript with boundless delight. If we were to publish your paper, it would be impossible for us to publish any work of a lower standard. And it is unthinkable that in the next thousand years we shall see its equal, we are, to our regret, etc. (cited in Fishman 2000, p. 129).

Criticism
Expect that not everyone will agree with or like your work once it is published. Criticism is inevitable. It is important to remember, however, that criticism in the form of *disagreement*, *disputation* and *debate* is the *beginning* of our thinking, not its end, and can provide rich fodder for future works. The whole field of philosophy has rested on this premise for centuries and would not have developed to the stage that it has today were it not for a healthy regard for, and acceptance of, the role of disagreement, disputation and debate in stimulating thought and generating reasoned and defensible arguments for and against certain propositions.

So long as criticism of your work is given within the spirit and legitimate boundaries of academic critique, it can serve the purpose of stimulating further thinking on your subject and of even bringing your work to the attention of a wider audience. What is crucial is *how* the criticism and disagreement is expressed. Obviously, criticism that is personally derogatory or attacks the person rather than the ideas, or which seriously misrepresents a writer's work, is neither appropriate nor acceptable, and may even be libellous. It is understandable that a writer would feel hurt and affronted by a personalised attack or a misleading and fraudulent representation of his or her work. Should this happen to you, always respond with dignity, not in kind. Depending on the seriousness of a criticism (especially if it is defamatory) your options are to either:

- ignore the criticism (thereby denying it the kudos of being worthy of attention)
- publish a patient and considered response to the criticism, pointing out the errors that your critic has made in reading and (mis)representing your work
- place the matter in the hands of your legal representative for mediation and resolution.

Arguably, a more challenging situation for an author is to have his or her work *completely ignored* by critics or other writers in the field. Being ignored, paradoxically, is probably the worst criticism of all since it seems to be saying: *your work is not even worthy of notice, not worthy of attention.*

Redundancy

If you are the author of a book (or books), expect that there will come a time when your work is no longer purchased, photocopied or cited. Academic books have a relatively short shelflife. The world and contexts in which scientific and practice knowledge is developed is constantly changing and so it is inevitable that, with time, professional literature once considered to be cutting edge will lose its currency and be regarded as out of date.

Only a very small percentage of academic books stay in print beyond their first print run (that is, are either reprinted as a first edition, or as subsequent revised editions). Once the sales of a book drop below a financially sustainable level, it is no longer a viable business proposition for a commercial publisher. The publisher's options (and contractual rights) are to either let the book go out of print, or to decisively withdraw the book from the market and either pulp any remaining copies or remainder what few copies are left at a discount. When this happens, and a publisher notifies you that it has decided not to reprint your book, it is important that you *do not take it personally*. As disappointing as it can be, this is an entirely normal and expected course of events.

Once a book goes out of print, the copyright in the work is normally returned to the author. This means that the author is free to republish the work in whatever form he or she wishes and may approach another company to have the work published as it stands or as a revised edition.

POLITICS OF ENVY

When you achieve success as an author (and even when you get your first article or book published), understand that not everybody will be as happy and excited as you and your advocates about you having achieved your writing goals. Unfortunately, people (including those with whom we work closely) do not always respond appropriately or in ways that we might expect in the event of our own or another's scholarly achievements. If your achievements have been the subject of public praise or attention, ironically this can give rise to what Susan Mitchell (2000, p. 98) calls 'the politics of envy'. Reflecting on her own experience as a successful author, newspaper columnist and broadcaster, Mitchell writes:

> When I published my first book, *Tall Poppies*, it became an immediate best-seller. I expected foolishly that my colleagues and, more importantly, my supervisors in the university would be pleased for me and for the reflected success on the institution. Instead, I found not only stony silence on the topic but snide remarks about becoming rich on the book's royalties. And with each successive and successful book, a slow realisation dawned on me that far from being praised for my success in the outside world, I was being punished for it inside the academic world . . . The unspoken view was that I had received more than my fair share of recognition and praise. My public profile for an academic was already too high.
>
> It took me a long time to come to terms with the fact that my academic colleagues would never give me any recognition for my work.

Mitchell (2000, p. 99) cites the examples of other successful authors, including the English writer C.S. Lewis and the Australian playwright David Williamson, who have become the targets of envy on account of their success. Williamson, for example, is reported as admitting that he 'never experienced real vitriol until he became publicly successful in Australia'.

Mitchell (2000, p. 98) contends that 'Public praise, whatever form it takes, will often bring people in conflict with other people'. Hidden at the base of this conflict, she suggests, is *envy*. On the question of how do deal with the politics of envy, the short answer is simply: *ignore it.* Regain your focus and get on with the business of writing and furthering your career as a successful author (see also the discussion on 'Envy' and strategies for dealing with it in Page, 1998, pp. 194–202).

BE PROFESSIONAL

It is important to treat writing as a profession, and for writers to behave like professionals and to present a professional image in the course of their work.

A professional image is best promoted:

- *in person* by displaying 'good manners' and observing the rules of common courtesy; being respectful; being reliable, such as by attending appointments on time, responding to phone/email/fax messages promptly, submitting manuscripts on or before specified time-lines; and communicating in an approachable and engaging manner

- *on paper* by using business cards; using letterhead paper for correspondence; following the conventions of letter writing; using quality paper (white bond photocopy stock); using an up-to-date curriculum vitae/resume that is well set out and portrays you as a credible author and someone who is worth investing in; supplying a head-and-shoulders photograph (for some journals); presenting manuscripts that comply with author guidelines.

Keeping track of your work and ensuring that you do not 'double up' can also enhance your professional image as a writer. To avoid doubling up, keep a record of:

- industry contacts (for example, acquisition/managing editors, book representatives)
- phone calls and correspondence to prospective publishers
- material/manuscripts sent out
- who material/manuscripts were sent to
- when they were sent
- by what date a reply is expected and the date a reply is received
- why, in the event of rejection, a submission is rejected (Day 1993).

HAVE A PLACE TO WRITE

To write effectively it is critical that you have a designated space to work. Having a designated writing space (that is, your own writing desk and preferably a study or an office) is just as critical to disciplined writing as is working to a writing schedule. As the English novelist and essayist Virginia Woolf wrote so famously in 1929, 'a woman must have . . . a room of her own if she is to write' (Woolf 1945, p. 6). This advice applies, of course, to all writers. Having a room of your own means that you can have somewhere to go and that, upon entering that domain, you can 'shut the door'—even if it is only for a few hours—and focus entirely on your writing.

DEVELOP MOMENTUM

Develop momentum as a writer and let the force of this momentum do its work. Describing the nature and importance of momentum, Du Mu counsels in Sun Tzu's *The art of war*, 'Roll rocks down a ten-thousand-foot mountain, and they cannot be stopped—this is because of the mountain, not the rocks' (Translated by Thomas Cleary (1988), p. 99).

Success often takes on a life of its own; once achieved, like rocks rolling down a mountain side, it cannot be stopped. As motivational literature is fond of pointing out, 'success breeds success'—that's momentum.

SUMMARY

Writing needs to be approached in a professional and disciplined manner. In order to develop a successful writing career, writers must first *want* to write and should focus primarily on writing about what they know and what is of interest to them. Writers need also to remember that writing and developing a good writing style takes time, practice and patience. Reading prolifically and attentively, having a good reference library and other resource materials, getting constructive feedback from others, being a 'self-mentor', being prepared to accept the lows as well as the highs of writing and publishing and maintaining momentum are all critical to achieving one's writing goals.

Equally important to a writer's success is finding an ally reader to support them on their writer's journey. An ally reader is someone who can be trusted:

- personally—will have the writer's interests at heart
- professionally—has integrity and won't abuse the support relationship to his/her own professional advantage
- emotionally—will not destroy the writer with unconstructive criticism (note, because of the intensely personal nature of authorship, the craft of writing is an emotionally sensitive process; a writer can thus be made or broken by an insensitive and harsh critic)
- intellectually—is competent academically and a 'good thinker'.

EXERCISES

1. Outline what winning habits you have and what habits you need to develop if you are to succeed as an author.
2. Prepare a plan for your writing career.

5 | PRODUCING A WORK

'Decide what you want to do. Then decide to do it. Then do it.'

—Zinsser (1998, p. 285)

'One of the wisest uses of time is to think about precisely what it is that you wish or need to say.'

—Manser and Curtis (2002, p. 185)

Once you have formulated your mission as a writer, prepared your writing schedule and attended to the 'environmental' issues of writing space, writing tools, and so forth, there comes the task of actually crafting a piece of work—the doing.

Regardless of your field, the topic you are writing on, the level at which you are writing, the proposed length of the work, your intended audience or your publishing timelines, the act of writing fundamentally involves the following active processes:

1. generating ideas and choosing a topic
2. being clear about what you are setting out to do

3. researching thoroughly and reading widely about the subject
4. examining carefully both your own and others' thinking on the subject
5. allowing your ideas to grow and take shape
6. formulating an outline of what you are going to write
7. engaging in the physical act of writing, structuring the work and preparing a first draft
8. reviewing and revising the first draft (and where relevant, subsequent drafts) of the work
9. deciding to stop
10. completing the final copy of the work
11. submitting the work for peer review and publication.

THE ACTIVE PROCESS OF WRITING

A good way to make a start and to begin writing productively is to write a critical commentary or an opinion piece on an issue about which you feel strongly and in which you would like others to become interested and to take action. In pursuing this option, it is important to remember that not all 'good' writing is or has to be the kind of *scholarly* writing that is generally written exclusively for academic journals and texts. Some very good writing can also be done for and is found in, for example, the commentary sections of professional journals and other related mass-circulation media (for example, campus and industry magazines and newspapers like *Campus Review*). Mass-circulation media outlets are always looking for material and are generally receptive to receiving good short articles. The question is: how to start?

Writing a persuasive commentary, editorial or opinion piece

Writing in health care domains is not just about communicating ideas; it is also fundamentally about persuading people to accept those ideas and, where applicable, to act on them to achieve some practical purpose. If writing in health professional contexts were not about questioning and challenging the status quo and 'making a difference', there would be little point to it.

Peter Thompson (1998, p. 5) explains that one of the great masters of persuasive communication was the ancient Greek philosopher, Aristotle. Indeed, Aristotle's principles of persuasive speech or rhetoric continue to be taught today and 'remain the foundations of modern persuasion'.

According to Aristotle, people can be persuaded by direct evidence or by the use of:

- *ethos* (a speaker's character)
- *logos* (a speaker's reasoned argument)
- *pathos* (the speaker's passion) (Thompson 1998, p. 7).

More simply, as Thompson (1998, p. 8) explains, 'being persuasive is really about speaking from your heart, your head and your soul'. Drawing on Aristotle's principles of rhetoric, Thompson (1998, pp. 18–19) believes that the key to persuasive communication is to structure a speech or a presentation according to the following prototype five-point plan:

1. *Bait (exordium)*: A story or statement which arouses audience interest.

2. *Problem or question (narratio)*: You pose a problem or question that has to be solved or answered.
3. *Solution or answer (confirmatio/probatio)*: You resolve the issues which have been raised.
4. *Pay-off or benefit (peroration)*: You state specific advantages to each member of the audience of adopting the course of action recommended in the solution or answer.
5. *Call to action (peroratio)*: You state the concrete actions which should follow your presentation.

An example of how this five-point plan could be used to structure and plan an article on a topic relevant to health care is as follows:

Topic: Patients' rights to informed consent and 'Do Not Attempt Resuscitation (DNAR)' directives
1. *Bait*: Patients in our public hospitals are being made the subjects of 'Do Not Attempt Resuscitation (DNAR)' directives without their knowledge or consent.
2. *Problem*: This situation involves a fundamental violation of patients' rights to be informed and to decide about their care and treatment options.
3. *Solution*: Policies and guidelines on the processes and procedures for prescribing and initiating DNAR directives need to be devised and implemented in the public hospital system.
4. *Pay-off*: Adopting sound DNAR policies and guidelines is good clinical risk management and will help to prevent the withholding or implementation of

resuscitation procedures against a patient's will, and spare the hospital and staff from becoming subject to serious complaint and possible litigation.

5. *Call to action*: Develop sound DNAR policies and guidelines for implementation in the public hospital system.

A useful variation of the five-point plan is Thompson's (1998, pp. 26–7) four-point plan, which is structured as follows:

1. *Situation*: The situation is designed to be a brief synopsis or overview of conditions that are already well known to the audience, which sets the focus of the article. Do not create disagreement at this stage.
2. *Complication*: Identify a complication or problem that threatens the viability of the status quo outlined in the situation. The complication may answer one of the following questions:
   - what's changed?
   - what's happened?
   - what's new?
   - what's different now?
   - what's upset the way things were?
   - what's gone wrong?
3. *Question*: The problem identified in the complication leads to the formation of a question. For example:
   - what can be done?
   - what choices do we have?
   - how can we succeed?
   - how do we proceed?

4. *Answer*: The answer or hypothesis takes up the bulk of the article and is a detailed response to the issue raised in the question.

An example of how this four-point plan could be used to structure and plan an article on a topic relevant to health care is as follows:

1. *Situation*: People suffering from mental illness and other mental health problems are among the most stigmatised, discriminated against, marginalised, disadvantaged and vulnerable members of society.
2. *Complication*: Although much has been done to improve the status quo, it is evident that a great deal more needs to be done to improve the plight of the mentally ill. Unless things are improved the mentally ill will continue to suffer a disproportionate burden of ill health and suffering which, in turn, will have an enormous cost (financial as well as human) for the community and society at large.
3. *Question*: What can be done to improve the status quo? What can be done to improve the plight of the mentally ill?
4. *Answer*: We need to overturn the pathology of prejudice and the stigma of difference that is interfering with processes for achieving social justice for the mentally ill. Specifically we need to:
   • 'take seriously the perspective of the mentally ill' (something that has not been the norm in the past)
   • expand the definition of 'who is the same, thus

challenging the exclusory uses of differences'; and
* broaden the definition of difference so that more traits (including previously devalued ones) 'become relevant to the distribution of a particular benefit' (adapted from Minow, 1990, pp. 95–6).

The content of this example has been drawn from an article I wrote after having had a personal experience that left me feeling disturbed about the degree to which people with mental illness are stigmatised and unjustly discriminated against (Johnstone 2001). Coincidentally, around the same time, I was invited to present a keynote address at an international conference for mental health nurses. I accepted the invitation and resolved to approach the task by writing a reflective commentary on the issue of stigma, social justice and the rights of the mentally ill. When writing this paper I unashamedly wrote with my 'head, my heart and my soul'.

I subsequently revised the paper and submitted it for publication. When the article was peer-reviewed, one of the reviewers expressed concern about it being more 'commentary' than scholarly in nature. Since the other reviewers' comments were favourable, however, the journal decided to accept the manuscript for publication and, in fact, published it as a feature article. Significantly, I received more responses from readers to this article than to any of my other works. Shortly after the article was published I received emails, faxes and surface mail from readers (including psychiatrists, psychologists, psychotherapists, mental health nurses and consumers) in Australia, Switzerland, Singapore, India, Canada and

New Zealand, requesting reprints of the article and thanking me for the work. Most of those who corresponded with me indicated that the article was very helpful to their clients and that they would recommend the article to future clients. Two psychiatrists indicated they would be using the article for teaching purposes. The work had achieved its intended purpose: it had made a difference to the lives of others (notably clients).

Whether using the five-point or four-point plan, if a work is to achieve its purpose, discussion will need to be informed by reliable references, examples and quotes and will need to exhibit all the principles of style. It is not enough just to write to a plan; as with any other writing, it is also necessary to have a thorough knowledge and understanding of the subject matter in order to be able to put a plan to effective use.

Writing scholarly philosophic works

Another way of developing your writing career is to write critical or scholarly philosophic articles on a subject. Scholarly philosophic writing has a rich and distinctive history dating back to ancient times and is commonly used in the fields of philosophy, theology and law. A good example of scholarly work can be found in the influential philosophic works of the ancient Greek philosophers Plato (c.428–c.348 BC) and Aristotle (384–22 BC); the works of these philosophers have survived to this day and remain in print in different language translations around the world.

Despite its rich, distinctive and credible history, philosophic writing and scholarship is sometimes misunderstood in health care domains and treated as being less credible than, say, writing that has as its focus the presentation of empirical (hands-on) research. I know of at least one occasion in which a scholarly philosophic article was rejected by the editor of a professional journal on grounds that, in her view and the view of its reviewers, it was 'too subjective'; the erroneous reasoning behind this judgement was that the article did not contain any 'facts'. This kind of reasoning is, unfortunately, not uncommon among editors and researchers unfamiliar with the tenets of philosophic inquiry. For this reason it would be worthwhile here to explain a little about what philosophic inquiry is and the nature of scholarly philosophic writing.

The tenets of philosophic inquiry and scholarly writing

It is generally recognised within the field of analytical philosophy that a substantial portion of philosophic inquiry is scholarly research. Some knowledge cannot be discovered or developed by empirical research. As the North American philosopher Thomas Nagel (1987, p. 4) explains:

> Philosophy is different from science and from mathematics. Unlike science it doesn't rely on experiments or observations, but only on thought. And unlike mathematics it has no formal methods of proof. It is done just by asking questions, arguing, trying out ideas and thinking of possible arguments against them, and wondering how our concepts really work.

Philosophic inquiry is appropriate for generating new knowledge not obtainable via empirical research. Unlike empirical research, however, philosophic inquiry has no distinctive method (Nielsen 1987, p. 16; Emmet 1968, p. 20; Edgerton 1988, p. 169). If there is a method peculiar to philosophy, it is fundamentally that 'of stating one's problem clearly and of examining its various proposed solutions critically' (Emmet 1968, p. 20). This, in turn, involves the 'development of various forms of intellectual analyses and arguments' (Edgerton 1988, p. 169). Thus, quoting again from Thomas Nagel (1987, pp. 4–5):

> The center of philosophy lies in certain questions which the reflective human mind finds naturally puzzling, and the best way to begin the study of philosophy is to think about them directly . . . The main concern of philosophy is to question and understand very common ideas that all of us use every day without thinking about them. A historian may ask what happened at some time in the past, but a philosopher will ask, 'What is time?' A mathematician may investigate the relations among numbers, but a philosopher will ask, 'What is a number?' . . . Anyone can ask whether it's wrong to sneak into a movie without paying, but a philosopher will ask, 'What makes an action right or wrong?'

The structure of a scholarly philosophic work
Writing a philosophic work essentially involves writing a defence thesis. The word *thesis* is a Greek word that

literally means 'a thing placed'. In the case of a defence thesis, the thing placed is a *proposition*.

Writing a defence thesis provides writers with a wonderful opportunity to take a stand or a position on something, and to develop their ideas in a focused, systematic, thorough and precise way (Seech 1997). Although the ultimate aim is to show there are better reasons for accepting than rejecting the position taken, philosophic writing is generally regarded as being more substantive than mere rhetoric (as discussed earlier), the main difference being that *persuasion* is achieved by carefully considered and reasoned (sound and logical) argument and counterargument, not 'overblown rhetoric' (Seech 1997, p. 14).

Scholarly philosophic writing is, by its nature, *argumentative*. It begins with a proposition and then proceeds by expounding 'arguments' in defence of the claim. This process tends to include the articulation not only of arguments *for* the proposition, but the consideration of and response to possible counter-arguments to the views expressed. Although it may not be possible to 'prove' a defence thesis, the writer can nevertheless provide good reasons why a clear-thinking person ought to accept them (Seech 1997; Nagel 1987; van Hooft et al. 1995).

In scholarly philosophic work, the thesis or proposition is really an 'ultimate conclusion'; and the body of the discussion is really the 'body of evidence' supporting that conclusion (Seech 1997, p. 15). This body of evidence is comprised primarily of literature sources as well as 'thought experiments' and reasoned arguments.

It should be noted that the term 'argument' as used in

philosophic inquiry has a discipline-specific meaning. Specifically, a philosophic argument is 'a linked set of statements [premises] designed to lead to a conclusion' (van Hooft et al. 1995, p. 36). For a conclusion to be valid it must follow from its premises. In the following example, for instance, you can see that the conclusion 'Socrates is mortal' is fundamentally linked to and follows directly from the premises that 'All men are mortal' and that 'Socrates is a man':

Premise 1:   All men are mortal.
Premise 2:   Socrates is a man.
Conclusion: Socrates is mortal.

In order to 'collapse' an argument (by showing it to be false and thereby destroying the case) a critic would need to show (by providing evidence) either that the premises were false and/or that the conclusion does not follow from the premises. For example, in order to collapse the above argument, a critic would need to show that either:

1. not all men are mortal (present the example of even one man who is living forever)
2. Socrates is not a man (Socrates could, for example, be a fish)
3. Socrates is immortal (the conclusion doesn't follow from the premise, for example, where it has been shown that Socrates is not a man but a rare immortal fish).

Now to use a more realistic example, consider the following argument:

Premise 1: People should always have high fibre cereals for breakfast
Premise 2: X is a high fibre cereal
Conclusion: All people (including myself) should eat X for breakfast.

In order to collapse this argument, or to show that it is not 'true', a critic would need only to show (with scientific evidence) that:

Against premise 1: Not all people should, in fact, have high fibre cereals for breakfast (for example, those who are fasting and those who, for reasons of illness, cannot tolerate high fibre foods)
Against premise 2: X is not, in fact, a high fibre cereal (it may have been mistakenly thought to be a high fibre cereal)
Against the conclusion: It is not the case that all people (including myself) should eat X for breakfast.

Unfortunately it is not possible within the scope of this present work to provide an in-depth discussion on the elements, form, content and general nature of philosophic reasoning and argument, and its application in health care scholarship. These issues are discussed comprehensively in *Writing Philosophy Papers* by Zachary Seech (1997) and *Facts and Values: An introduction to critical thinking for nurses* by Stan van Hooft et al. (1995). In the space remaining, however, it is appropriate to outline the general structure of a philosophic work and dispel some of the popular misconceptions and misunderstandings that still surround scholarly philosophic writing in health care domains.

Like all writing, scholarly writing has a beginning, middle and an end. The opening paragraph to a scholarly work should state precisely the claim or 'point of contention' to be defended in the body of the work and include an outline of how it will be defended (van Hooft et al. 1995, pp. 54–68). The body of the work (the main discussion) should present the 'evidence' (arguments and counter arguments) supporting the point of contention. Finally, the conclusion should summarise what has been achieved. In essence, the conclusion should do little more than 'mirror' the opening paragraph: it should briefly restate the claim (point of contention), review the main arguments advanced in support of it, and generally confirm delivery of what was promised in the opening paragraph (Seech 1997, pp. 10–12). As a general rule, no *new* material should be introduced in the conclusion. If the ideas in a conclusion have not been defended in the body of the work, *they should not be included*.

Before commencing a scholarly work it is advisable to plan or outline the basic structure of your paper. Devising such a plan will help you to:

- focus, organise and order your thinking
- check and track the logic and coherency of the arguments you are planning to advance in support of your proposition
- help you to 'keep on track' and not get distracted by issues that are tangential to your topic (Seech 1997, p. 13).

Prototype plan for structuring a scholarly philosophic paper

The following is a prototype plan for structuring a scholarly philosophic paper.

1. *Opening paragraph*
   (a) Statement of the 'point of contention' or claim to be defended.
   (b) Outline of the main points or arguments to be advanced in support of the claim made:
      (i) point one (also serving as a 'signpost' to the first subheading)
      (ii) point two (also serving as a 'signpost' to the second subheading)
      (iii) point three (also serving as a 'signpost' to the third subheading).

2. *Body of the discussion*
   (a) First point (subheading).
   (b) Second point (subheading).
   (c) Third point (subheading).
   (*Note*: Discussion under the respective subheadings may be broken up under further sub-subheadings. Counterarguments can be presented as sub-subheadings under these points or under a separate subheading, whichever is appropriate).

3. *Conclusion*
   (a) Restatement of the point of contention.
   (b) Restatement of the mains points advanced in support of the point of contention:
      (i) point one
      (ii) point two
      (iii) point three.

An example of how this prototype plan might be used to outline the content and approach of an article on a specific health care topic is as follows:

Topic: Health professionals reported for the misconduct of child maltreatment: ethical issues for disciplinary panels

1. *Opening paragraph*
    (a) Point of contention: Regulating authorities should adopt a formal policy position of 'zero tolerance' towards health professionals found to have abused children and should impose the maximum penalty of deregistration in cases were allegations have been sustained.
    (b) Outline of the main points to be advanced in support of the claim made:
        (i) Child maltreatment is professional mis-conduct of a *serious nature at the upper end of seriousness.*
        (ii) Child maltreatment by health professionals constitutes a violation of conduct standards otherwise expected by the public.
        (iii) Regulating authorities have a primary obli-gation to protect the public interest, not the professionals who have offended against children.
        (iv) Misconduct of a serious nature at the upper end of seriousness warrants the most severest of sanctions: *deregistration.*

2. *Body of the discussion*
   (a) First subheading: Child maltreatment as professional misconduct of a serious nature.
       Sub-subheadings:
       (i)   The nature of child maltreatment
       (ii) The nature of professional misconduct
       (iii) The constituents of misconduct of a 'serious nature' at the 'upper end of seriousness'.
   (b) Second subheading: Professional conduct standards.
       Sub-subheadings:
       (i) Nature and purpose of professional conduct standards
       (ii) Standards of professional conduct expected by the public.
   (c) Third subheading: Health professional regulating authorities and protection of the public interest.
       Sub-subheadings:
       (i)   Protecting the public interest
       (ii) Public trust and protecting the good reputation and standing of the profession
       (iii) Professional misconduct of a serious nature and forfeiting the right to practice as a professional
       (iv) Nature and purpose of a 'zero tolerant' position
       (v)   Moral and professional imperatives of adopting a zero tolerant position and de-registering health professionals who have maltreated children.
3. *Conclusion*
   Regulating authorities have a responsibility to adopt a formal policy position of 'zero tolerance' towards

health professionals found to have abused children and impose the maximum penalty of deregistration in cases were allegations have been sustained. This is because:

(i) Child maltreatment is professional misconduct of a *serious nature*.

(ii) Child maltreatment by health professionals constitutes a violation of conduct standards otherwise expected by the public.

(iii) Regulating authorities have a primary obligation to protect the public interest, not the professionals who have offended against children.

(iv) By deregistering health professionals who have maltreated children, regulating authorities will send a message to the public and to the profession that the abuse of children is not acceptable and that health professionals have a special obligation to protect children and to take appropriate action when the interests of children are violated by people in a professional and trusted position (see Johnstone 1999b).

Writing empirical research articles

Writing an empirical research article, that is, an article in which the findings of either a quantitative or qualitative research study are presented, is arguably more straightforward than writing scholarly philosophic works. Depending on the journal in which the work is published, empirical research articles are generally structured as follows:

1. opening paragraph
2. background to the study
3. study design
4. study findings
5. discussion (incorporating a concluding paragraph).

Variations in this structure are usually slight, for example:

- For *qualitative* research studies
  1. introduction
  2. literature review
  3. theoretical framework (discussion of methodology)
  4. methods (discussion of steps/techniques)
  5. findings
  6. discussion (incorporating a concluding paragraph and recommendations).
- For *quantitative* research studies
  1. background to the study
  2. methods
  3. results
  4. discussion (incorporating a concluding paragraph and recommendations).

In either case, the opening paragraph usually contains a poignant opening sentence to 'hook' the reader. Unless there is a separate subheading signalling a discussion on the background to the study, the opening paragraph usually provides an overview of the research study including:

- information on the background to and rationale for the study

- the research question(s)
- the aims of the study.

Under the 'methods' subheading, attention is given to discussing:

- the theoretical underpinnings of the study
- the description of the sample
- the means of accessing the sample
- data collection and analysis
- limits of the study
- a statement confirming ethics approval and compliance with prescribed research ethics standards.

The presentation of results/findings and their discussion will depend on the nature of the study and, crucially, the word limit set by a receiving journal. Findings are usually presented and discussed in the form of a succinct synopsis rather than as an elaborate exhaustive narrative. In fact, within most journal articles there tends to be very little commentary on the results (Thomas 2000, p. 119). The discussion section provides a discussion of the answers to the research questions; if there is no sub-headed conclusion to the article, the discussion in this section generally concludes with a recommendation for further research and, where appropriate, a call for the practical application of the findings such as in the form of a practice or policy change. Statements in a conclusion are typically crafted along the lines of 'What should be done next?' (Thomas 2000, p.119).

Although the structure of empirical research articles

is less complicated than philosophic papers, writers still need to take care in crafting their work. As with any scholarship, the background to an empirical study, the processes used for undertaking the study and the study's findings all need to be presented and discussed in a logical, salient, coherent and defensible manner. The strategies of philosophic writing can be particularly helpful in this regard, particularly when providing a critical discussion of the findings. Even though the techniques of philosophic writing and reasoning are not the primary 'methods' used in empirical research articles, they have an important adjunct role to play nonetheless.

Where relevant, the use of tables and figures need to be pertinent and presented clearly in the article. (For a helpful discussion on how to present research findings concisely, coherently and clearly, see Thomas 2000, pp. 79–86.)

Writing for newsletters

Writing for newsletters can provide another valuable opportunity to develop your skills as a writer. Although newsletters tend to be informal in style, writing articles for inclusion in them should still be approached with diligence, discipline and care. A newsletter that is badly produced and contains 'bad' writing could prove a disaster for the organisation or group sponsoring it and the writers contributing to it.

The primary purpose of a newsletter is to promote communication between an organisation or a special interest group and its constituents. For example, the *RMIT Nursing Quarterly*, a quarterly newsletter produced by the Department of Nursing and Midwifery at RMIT University, has been produced to foster communication between the department and its:

- industry partners
- staff
- current students
- alumni
- other academic colleagues both within and outside of the university.

Other key purposes served by the production of a newsletter are to:

- *connect* with constituents and to foster in them a sense of community and belonging
- *inform* and keep constituents up to date with the latest happenings and issues of mutual interest
- *involve* constituents by giving them an opportunity to respond to and to participate in certain events and activities promoted in the newsletter (including contributing articles)
- *activate* constituents by putting out a 'call to action'.

Writing in newsletters tends to be *conversational* in style. In using a conversation style of writing, however, just as much attention needs to be paid to the elements and principles of style (see Chapter 3 of this book) as with scholarly and other creative non-fiction writing.

Successful newsletter writing and production have a number of features in common. In summary 'good' newsletter writing is:

- *current*—and preferably a 'step ahead' of other outlets
- *concise*—most contributions should normally be no longer than 350–400 words in length
- *accurate*—information contained in an article should be accurate, valid and reliable; if fraudulent or inappropriate claims are made in the material published this can be very damaging not only to the writer but also to the newsletter and to the organisation or group producing it
- *informative*—shares information that is of interest, is pertinent, and meets readers 'need to know' (adapted from Baverstock 2002, pp. 61–2).

GENERAL ADVICE ON PRODUCING A WORK

Whether writing for publication in a professional journal, a book, a newspaper or a newsletter, careful attention should always be paid to the following processes.

Choosing a title

Choosing a title for a work can be an exasperating experience for a writer. One day you might think you have the perfect title only to change your mind the next and deem it trivial and boring. Regardless, it is important that when you start writing an article or book you at least have a *working title* for the work. Once you have a working title, then you can start looking for the 'perfect title'—which can take some time. Susan Page (1998, p. 24) argues, controversially, that in your quest for the 'fabulous title', you should sit down and write no less than 30 titles in one sitting! Once you have a title and have a sense of 'eureka', ask others for their opinion and gauge their reactions.

The title of a work should:

- convey to the reader what the work is about
- provide this information at a glance (bearing in mind that readers often scan book shelves looking for titles relevant to their interests and will pick up only those that catch their eye)
- convince the reader the work is 'for them'.

According to Page (1998, p.18) a good title should accomplish most if not all of the following tasks:

- instantly say what the work is about
- pique our curiosity
- be distinctive
- be memorable
- be positive
- feel on target, exciting and compelling *to the author*.

I would add that the title should also be descriptive, not metaphorical, and contain key words that will ensure it is noticed and located in the appropriate citation indexes. For example, a paper entitled 'The tea-bag phenomenon' (which is about health research in action) will probably not be noticed as readily as it might otherwise be if it contained keys words more appropriate to its subject matter and content.

Other helpful tips in crafting a title are:

- avoid words that can be spelled in different ways
- make the title easy to remember
- avoid titles that begin with *How to* . . . (books in print contain over 6000 titles that begin with these words)
- include subtitles (these give you the chance to add more information to a title and to hook a potential reader (adapted from Page 1998, pp. 21–2).

Preparation

Critical to any writing process is the level of preparation that is undertaken before embarking on the work. Preparation includes not just undertaking a pertinent or exhaustive literature search and review, but also thinking deeply about the topic, being open to and exploring new ideas (from all manner of sources, including informal and incidental sources) and generally ordering your thoughts on the topic. It also involves deciding 'what single point you want to leave in the reader's mind' (Zinsser 1998, p. 53) and working diligently to uphold all the principles of style to enable you to make that point powerfully, impressively and persuasively.

The quality of a work will always depend on the quality of the information contained within it—whether it is accurate, pertinent, salient and complete—not merely on the manner of its presentation. A work could, for example, be technically perfect yet utterly lifeless and unimpressive. When preparing to write a work, search for, think about and collate information in a manner that ultimately leaves you feeling that 'no rock has been left unturned', and ensure the completed work leaves the reader with that feeling too.

Literature reviews

Sometimes writers preparing literature reviews for a research thesis or report write to show *what they have read*, rather than to 'sketch out for the reader the intellectual path that the writer has followed in order that readers may follow as well' (Rankin 2001, p. 42). When writing a literature review it is important that you consider whether the literature you have reviewed provides evidence for the points you are advancing. If not, do not include it in your final report/manuscript.

Writing an abstract

An abstract is a short summary or a condensed version of a piece of writing such as a journal article, research proposal or report (the journal abstract equivalent for a book is normally its Preface). An abstract may range in length from 50 to 300 words, depending on the publication or research application document in which it will appear.

Abstracts are commonly used in electronic abstract databases such as CINAHL and Medline, and hence are widely disseminated. When writing an abstract, it is important therefore to keep in mind its fundamental purpose, namely to allow other researchers to scan quickly through the latest professional publications to source information that is relevant to their work. For example, it is possible to scan up to 600 abstracts in a few hours when undertaking a literature search for a journal article or other publication. Being able to scan the abstracts over such a relatively short period of time (much shorter than it would take to read 600 articles) can speed up the research process and enable the writer to establish very quickly whether his or her thoughts, ideas and work are up to date, relevant, original and critical.

When crafting an abstract, the principles of Aristotle's rhetoric (see 'Writing a persuasive commentary, editorial or opinion piece' earlier in this chapter) apply since, in essence, you are trying to *sell* your article or report to prospective readers. The abstract should have a beginning, middle and an end, include key words, and provide a poignant snapshot of what the broader work is about. It may contain similar or even the same words used in an opening paragraph.

What you write will ultimately depend on the economy of words available to you. Whether writing 50 words or 300 words, however, extreme discipline—and style—is required.

Crafting the introduction

In several respects, the most important sentence and the most important paragraph of a work is the *first one*. This is because the first sentence and the paragraph that it leads into serves fundamentally as the 'hook' to prospective readers. If readers are not engaged immediately and if there is no incentive to read on, they will simply not continue.

When crafting your opening paragraph to a work, and the paragraphs following it, keep in mind the following principles:

- The lead sentence must capture the reader immediately.
- The lead 'must provide hard details that tell the reader

why the piece was written and why he [or she] ought to read it' (what's in it for them?).
- Coax the reader along the way.
- Tell a story.
- Add an element of surprise (for example, use something unexpected; the contrapuntal device can achieve this).
- When you are ready to stop, just stop (adapted from Zinsser 1998, pp. 55–67).

The use of headings and subheadings

Headings and subheadings are titles that serve to delineate subsections of a work. The main purpose of headings and subheadings is to provide 'signposts' to the reader so they know in which direction the information is heading.

In books, headings become the *table of contents* which can also serve as an 'easy find' index to the work (see, for example, the table of contents to this work). Writing out the headings and subheadings of a work (whether as a table of contents for a book, or as an outline for a journal article or book chapter) can give the writer an overall sense of the coherency of the work and where certain sections may need to be relocated to ensure a better progression of the ideas being advanced. To be effective, signposts, titles and subtitles need to be:

- clear about what is contained in the section or subsection
- short
- distinctive
- relevant (deliver what it says it will)

- eye-catching
- enticing to the reader.

The 'Matrioshka principle'

All works should have a clearly distinguishable beginning, middle and an end. In addition each subsection and sub-subsection of a work should likewise have a distinguishable beginning, middle and an end. It should be possible with a well-written piece of work to pick up any section of the work and, upon reading it, get a sense of and feel informed about both its parts as well as its whole. Like the classical Russian nesting doll (the *Matryoshka*, or the anglicised variant *Matrioshka*) which is characteristically comprised of *a doll nestling within a doll nestling within a doll*, and where each of the smaller dolls is a perfect or near-perfect replica of the immediate larger doll in which it is found, each subsection of a discussion should stand as a complete 'mini-discussion' in a larger work, that is, as *a discussion within a discussion within a discussion*. For teaching and writing purposes, I have called this the 'Matrioshka principle of writing'.

Unfettered writing

When embarking on your writing do not unduly limit or constrain yourself. Nothing can be more constraining to your creative thinking and writing than feeling fettered by a word limit or even by a writing plan. It is more productive to write freely and then radically edit a work to comply with a word limit, than to write tightly to a word limit from the beginning. Similarly, when writing to a plan it is better to exhaust your thoughts—even those that might be tangential to your work—than to constrain your thinking. Ideas and commentary that are tangential to your work can always be edited out later. In the interests of writing an innovative and benchmark work, 'Think broadly about your assignment . . . Push the boundaries of your subject and see where it takes you' (Zinsser 1998, p. 249). Engage freely in the writing process.

Staying on track

When writing it is always tempting to include and discuss issues that, while interesting, are not strictly relevant to the key point or points you are trying to make and emphasise. An important and general rule for writers is: *keep on track*. To assist you in deciding what is and what is not strictly relevant, apply the following rule: *if the information and/or references you are considering provide necessary support or background to a point you are trying to make, then include the material; if not, exclude it.*

Crafting the conclusion

Crucial to any writing is deciding where, when and how to conclude it. Often a work 'will tell you where it wants to stop', in that the ending just 'feels right' (Zinsser 1998, p. 283). When the ending comes, it is always important that readers have something to 'go away with'.

Pay careful attention to crafting the conclusions of your work. Just as the first sentence should function as a hook to *read on*, the last sentence should also function as a hook to read further on the subject, to take action or to recommend the work to others. Finish on an inspiring note. At the very least, leave the reader with a sense that the work and its conclusion were worth reading. Better still leave the reader with a powerful idea, an image, a taste, a desire to question and to act.

Bibliographies and reference lists

Novice writers are sometimes confused about the nature, purpose and the differences between a bibliography and a reference list, and which they should use. Your decision to use a reference list or a bibliography will have as much to do with the conventions and editorial requirements of a journal or publisher, as it will with your own personal preference. Most journals require reference lists; some journals also prescribe an upper limit on the number of references that can be used. In the case of book publishing, depending on word-limit requirements, some may advocate the use of either a reference list or a bibliography, or a combination of both.

The essential difference between a reference list and a bibliography is as follows:

- a *reference list* includes only those works that have been *quoted directly* in the text of a work
- a *bibliography* includes all works that have been *consulted* or *read* during the course of writing the text, including those that have *not* been quoted from directly.

When deciding whether to include a reference list or a bibliography in your publications, consider the following:

- the purpose of either a reference list or a bibliography is to leave an 'audit trail' so that readers can locate and gain access to the original works to which you have referred in the body of your work
- *always* include a full list of the works you have quoted from or used in preparing your publication
- including an accurate list of all the works you have read and which have influenced and/or informed your writing, assures readers of the integrity of your work and protects you against committing plagiarism
- editorial requirements and prescribed word limits may limit your options: you may have to include *either* a bibliography *or* a reference list depending on what has been prescribed by the publisher.

SUMMARY

Producing a work for publication (whether a journal article, a book, a newspaper commentary or an item for a newsletter) requires careful planning and thought. It also requires disciplined attention to drafting, redrafting and conducting a final edit of the work before submitting it for publication. Deciding when to stop can sometimes be as difficult as getting started. Often, however, the work draws to a 'natural' conclusion leaving the writer with a feeling of 'Ah, ha—that's it! It's finished!'.

EXERCISES

1. With reference to Thompson's five-point or four-point plan (see pages 93–8), write a persuasive commentary on a professional issue that is presently of concern to you and your colleagues.
2. Submit your commentary for publication in an appropriate professional journal or other publication.
3. Based on your commentary, prepare a plan for writing a scholarly article on the issue.
4. Share your commentary and writing plan with your mentor for feedback.
5. Commence researching and reviewing the literature in preparation for writing your scholarly article.
6. Set a writing schedule and commence writing the article.
7. Upon completion, submit the manuscript to an appropriate journal for review and publication.

6 | TROUBLESHOOTING

'. . . all writers face similar challenges. Whether they are writing a journal article or a grant proposal, a curriculum guide or a consultant's report, the writers in our faculty writing groups tend to raise the same questions, encounter the same obstacles, and offer the same kind of writing advice.'
—Rankin (2001, p. xii)

'People don't realise that being a writer is like climbing not one mountain but a whole range of mountains, and there's a higher range behind that, and a range behind that.'
—McAlpine (2000b, p. 63)

During the writing process all writers, both novice and experienced, will encounter difficulties of one kind or another. As Elizabeth Rankin (2001, p. 1) observes:

> Like all demanding professional work, writing keeps confronting us with new situations and challenges. In the process of negotiating these situations, we encounter complex ideas, multifaceted problems, and difficulties we have not dealt with before.

Whether the difficulties encountered are to be regarded as 'serious' will depend largely on the extent to which they:

- interfere with, impede or obstruct the writing process
- delay unacceptably or even prevent a work from being completed and published, not only on time but at all.

How well writers deal with the problems they encounter will often depend on their character, how creative they are, how disciplined their thinking is and how willing and able they are to engage constructively with those 'who share their interests and with those who challenge their assumptions' (Rankin 2001, p. 1).

While there is no magic recipe for dealing with the various difficulties that writers will inevitably encounter during the course of their writing careers, there are nevertheless some strategies that can be utilised to help prevent some of the more common types of difficulties from occurring or at least minimise their impact should they occur. One strategy is to know about the kinds of problems that can occur, anticipate them at the outset and have strategies in place to deal with them if and when they are encountered. The following are some examples.

GENERATING IDEAS

For some writers, particularly novice writers, the most difficult task is deciding what to write on and how to generate ideas. Difficulties can be encountered not just in finding topics to write on, but also in generating enough ideas to sustain the writing itself. In contrast, experienced writers may never be short of ideas, and are instead faced with the challenge of how to recognise and choose the most salient ideas for their work.

There are a number of strategies that can be used for generating ideas, such as those I've summarised below:

1. Be curious, and learn to *recognise ideas*. Ideas are scattered everywhere, not just in conventional sources (such as libraries, academic books and journal articles); look for ideas/material everywhere, for example, in
   - your surveillance of the world/work place
   - newspapers/magazines/mass-circulation media
   - visual arts—especially film
   - conversations (both formal and informal)
   - your social network (family/friends)
   - yourself (for example, personal experiences, responses to the human condition, political outrage)
   - your own publications—'In the body of every article you write lurk the seeds of several more' (Holmes 1969, p. 20)
   - the publications of others (adapted from Holmes 1969, pp. 11–21; Zinsser 1998, pp. 59, 253, 284; van Hooft et al. 1995; Ruggiero 1995).
2. Always collect more material than you will use. If something attracts your attention, collect it even if you are not sure how or if you will use it. There is nothing quite so frustrating as writing a work and suddenly remembering an anecdote or a quote or a reference, but not remembering its source or how to locate it.
3. Write down your ideas immediately: *keep a notebook and use it*. Then, using the ideas you have noted down, just sit down and *write* (Zinsser 1998).

OVERCOMING WRITER'S BLOCK

'Writer's block' is a colloquial term that is used to describe a situation in which a writer cannot think, cannot write and, as a result, cannot move forward in the writing process. It is, quite simply, a dreadful situation in which a writer finds himself/herself 'stuck' and which, paradoxically, sees the writer spending a large amount of writing time and energy '*not* writing' (Elbow 1998, p. 14).

Writer's block can occur at any time during the writing process: in the beginning, the middle and/or at the end of a work. Both inexperienced and experienced writers can experience it.

The causes of writer's block are many, and include:

- lack of confidence—lacking belief in one's own ability to produce the work
- fear—of producing a substandard work and what others might think about it (the fear of producing 'nothing but rubbish')
- panic—about a looming deadline and whether the work will be completed on time
- perfectionism—desire to produce a word-perfect draft/copy on the first attempt
- exhaustion—from working too hard at your usual job and literally being depleted of the energy to think and write.

The best way to overcome writer's block is to:

- avoid being judgemental about the situation and about yourself (accept that it 'just is', and that it will pass)

- avoid censuring or trivialising your work (this is being judgemental and will serve only to further cement your sense of being stuck and your procrastination)
- engage in 'freewriting' (no matter how 'blocked' you are feeling, sit down and write without stopping for ten minutes; it doesn't matter if the writing is good or bad since the whole point of this exercise is *to get writing* and to overcome the block in the process (see 'Freewriting' in Elbow 1998, pp. 13–19)
- resume the writing project: *get on with it.*

If you are exhausted, all that you may need is some 'space', that is, a short rest and a temporary break away from the writing process. Sometimes just going for a 20-minute walk can refresh and reinvigorate you. Whatever you decide to do, ensure that you resume writing as soon as possible so that you can get back on track.

DEALING WITH PROCRASTINATION

Procrastination is a form of writer's block and, unresolved, can be just as destructive to the writing process as full-blown writer's block. The causes of procrastination are similar to those that cause writer's block: lack of confidence, fear, perfectionism, exhaustion and overwork.

The best way to deal with procrastination is to:

- avoid being judgemental about the situation and about yourself (accept that every writer experiences procrastination at some stage during the writing

process and that it will pass; say to yourself in a matter of fact way, 'That's me—procrastinating', and let go)
- write a list of the things that you are putting off
- examine the list and assign a priority value to each task, putting the most important first, and the least important last (sometimes, however, starting on and completing a small though unimportant task, like adding a couple of references to your bibliography, can help to break the mood of procrastination since it is one less thing on the list that needs to be done and may be just enough to lessen the 'pressure cooker effect' that is stalling you in your work)
- focus on undertaking the most important and most urgent task first
- take one step at a time; as Vin Maskell and Gina Perry (1999, p. 165) advise:

> Don't allow yourself to feel overwhelmed by the extent of the task—break it down into a series of small steps. Keep each step simple and achievable. Take one step at a time and reward yourself as you complete each step.

- seek assistance (if the task is too difficult, or you have other tasks pressing that others could do, negotiate for some help)
- start writing (putting off the task does not get it done; furthermore, the longer you put it off, the bigger the task seems and the more overwhelming it becomes).

BENEFITS AND CHALLENGES OF CO-AUTHORSHIP

In many academic and professional circles, collaborative writing and co-authorship is the norm not the exception—

although, in nursing, the incidence of single-author papers tends to be higher relative to other health care/biomedical disciplines (Rafferty et al. 2000, p. 24). Collaborating with other authors both within and outside of your field or discipline can have many benefits, and when one is invited to collaborate on a work it can feel like a great honour—especially if the invitation has been extended to you in recognition of your standing in the field. Collaborative writing can also pose many challenges and when one is faced with some of those challenges, it can feel like a great burden.

One of the key benefits of author-collaboration is the sharing of discipline-specific knowledge and experience in a manner that enables:

- the development of new ideas and alternative perspectives on a subject
- improved and deeper understanding of a subject
- the creation of 'new knowledge'
- the development of innovative and productive connections between different and related subject matter
- finding new solutions to old problems, and new solutions to new problems
- bridging the gap between theory and practice (particularly in the case of academic–clinician collaborations)
- mentorship of inexperienced writers by experienced authors
- personal development (including the development of interpersonal skills and learning to work productively with others)
- professional development (not least developing multi-disciplinary skills outside of the knowledge and experience of your own discipline).

Another benefit of collaborative writing is that, in the sense of 'many hands make light work', it shares the burden of writing and producing publications to meet academic performance indicators. For instance, collaborating with a team of three or four authors and rotating the primary and associate author responsibilities to reflect the degree of each author's contribution to a work could result in an author participating in three or four peer-reviewed articles per year, instead of just one. Likewise with publishing larger works such as books. A book of twelve chapters written respectively by twelve authors or cooperatively with three collaborating authors is less onerous and arguably more manageable in a busy academic year than publishing a book of twelve chapters written by just one author.

Writing collaboratively also brings with it certain challenges. Collaborative writing can become particularly demanding when disagreement and conflict arises between participating authors. Disagreements and conflicts can occur even when a writing plan has been devised collaboratively and agreed upon before the project has begun. This is because, as Elizabeth Rankin (2001, p. 22) explains, most writers do their thinking and writing simultaneously and are often 'unable to know what they think until they see what they say'. In other words, it is not until a writer actually sits down and writes that it becomes clear what it is they are thinking and where their ideas are leading to. Thus, it is not until collaborating writers start their work and share their writing with each other that differences become evident in their:

- intellectual standpoints
- writing skills (in some instances, it may even become evident that a collaborating writer cannot write well)

- writing styles
- work habits
- attitudes toward the work
- priorities assigned to the work
- personalities.

In extreme cases, these differences can result in the authors moving in different directions, to the serious detriment of the work. Sometimes this can happen even when the collaborating authors have agreed to work with each other on the basis of 'knowing each other' and 'knowing each other's work' prior to the commencement of the collaborative project.

Dealing with disagreement and conflict between collaborating authors can be both difficult and stressful, particularly if it is impeding the progress of the work and the team's ability to meet the contractual timeline for the delivery of the completed manuscript. Professional relationships and reputations are also at stake. For these reasons it is imperative that conflicts between collaborating authors are resolved quickly and professionally. Strategies for preventing and dealing with a possible breakdown in author-collaborations include:

1. *Choose your co-authorship team carefully in the first place*: remember, we often do not know the people we work with as well as we think, and it is not until we work *closely* with them that we discover their true character and capabilities; remember also that the nature of a person's published work may not necessarily reflect how difficult or easy they are to work

with as a collaborating author (this applies whether you are the author inviting collaboration or you have been invited to collaborate with another author).

2. *Complete a detailed plan of the project before commencement of the work:* ensure that all co-participating authors are informed about, are clear about, understand and agree on the subject of the work, rationale for writing it, aims and objectives, intended audience, special features and characteristics that would distinguish the work from other similar works, word limits, timelines, and each author's specific rights, duties and responsibilities in regard to the work (*note*: it is wise and in some institutions a mandatory requirement to sign an 'authors agreement' form before commencing a work; this agreement should clarify issues such as intellectual property rights, author responsibilities, and so forth—much like a book contract).

3. *Act quickly and decisively to resolve conflict*: if and when there is so much as a *hint* of divisive differences emerging between the authors, work collectively, collaboratively and professionally to resolve these differences *as soon as possible*; differences that are allowed to fester can become irreconcilable and can place both the team and the work in jeopardy.

4. *Have a back-up plan*: sometimes the differences between one or more authors can become irreconcilable and it might be better, on the basis of a 'cost–benefit' analysis, for the disgruntled author/ authors to withdraw from the project; in the event of this happening make provisions for the writing responsibilities to be shared, where able, among the

remaining authors or engage a replacement author to carry out the work.

5. *Learn from the experience*: in the event of an author-collaboration breaking down, conduct a 'root cause' analysis of what went wrong and use the learning gained from conducting this analysis to inform the development and conduct of future collaborative projects.

PROMISES AND PERILS OF COMMISSIONED WRITING

On occasion a health professional or academic might be commissioned by a professional organisation, a government department, an independent publisher or some other entity to produce a 'special work' such as a book, a manual or a report on a designated topic, for a clearly specified purpose and for a specific audience. Receiving a commission of this nature is an honour since usually only people with international standing in their field are invited to take up such commissions. The benefits of undertaking commissioned work include:

- the kudos of being asked to undertake the work
- a unique opportunity to make a significant contribution of knowledge to the field
- further recognition for your work
- a unique opportunity to have an impact on the world (especially if the work is being commissioned to inform and improve policy and practice)
- personal and professional development
- an opportunity to demonstrate your capabilities and to fulfil job performance criteria.

Commissioned work is not, however, without its challenges. One of the biggest challenges is that often the parameters of the work are specified beforehand by the organisation or institution commissioning the work, leaving the author with little scope for using his or her professional discretion in deciding who to collaborate with (in the event of co-authored commissioned work), the content and structure of the work, and how and to whom, if at all, it will be presented. Ultimately, those who have commissioned the work have the final say on how, and if, the work will be used. These and related challenges are best dealt with preventatively, rather than remedially, such as by:

- *being clear about what is involved in undertaking a commissioned work and what is expected of you before accepting an invitation to do it.* In particular, clarify the:
  —subject matter
  —rationale for writing the work (why has it been commissioned?)
  —purpose, aims and objectives of the work
  —intended audience
  —how the work will be distributed/findings disseminated
  —how the work will be used
  —author rights and responsibilities (including issues of intellectual copyright, author acknowledgement [do not assume that your name will be on the cover], copy-editing resources and production standards, processes for dispute resolution, word limit and timelines)

—credentials, experience and reputation of other participating co-authors (where relevant)

- *ascertaining whether you agree generally with the scope of the work, including its purpose, aims and objectives* (if there is no room for negotiation and you have moral qualms about what is being requested and/or are ideologically opposed to what is being commissioned, DO NOT DO IT; remember: *what can look like a missed opportunity often is not*)

- *clarifying your availability and commitment to undertaking the work* (if you have other pressing commitments that may interfere with your ability to produce the work on time and at the standard expected, or your heart is not in it, you should seriously consider *not* accepting the invitation; beware: *failure is not an option*)

- *having a back-up plan* (in the event that you do find yourself commissioned and engaged in a work that is proving problematic, consult immediately with the commissioning body and seek to negotiate a solution to the problems being experienced; due to the mutual vested interests in the work, mutually agreeable solutions can usually be found).

CHALLENGES OF CONVERTING ASSIGNMENTS AND THESES INTO PUBLICATIONS

Students and colleagues sometimes ask whether an essay, an assignment or a minor thesis written for the purposes of fulfilling the assessment requirements of a university or professional development course is suitable for publication. The conventional view on this issue is that, in most instances, assignments written for the purposes of assessment are *not* suitable for publication—at least not unless they are substantially revised. The reasoning behind this view is that assignments of this nature (including minor theses) are generally written 'to show what we know' rather than 'to make a significant contribution of knowledge to the field' (Rankin 2001, p. 2).

In contradistinction to the nature and purpose of academic and professional writing, it is commonly assumed and understood that coursework assignments are:

- generally written for the purposes of enabling the writer to demonstrate to a teacher/examiner his or her *intellectual development*, not to participate in ongoing professional conversations on a given topic
- intended for only *one* reader (the teacher) or in the case of minor theses (one or two examiners), not a broader professional audience
- designed to assist in the development of writing skills for future academic and professional writing, not to expand interest in a subject and provide scholarly leadership in the field
- not readily transferable to suit the purposes of another context (such as publication), at least not without modification (Rankin 2001, pp. 2–3).

These assumptions should, however, be viewed with caution. My own view is that an assignment, essay or a minor thesis should not be dismissed as being unsuitable for publication *just because* it has been written for the purposes of formal assessment in a university or a professional development course. This is particularly so in the case of assignments that have been written on a 'free topic' and where the writers (often postgraduate students with considerable professional practice experience) have been encouraged to write on a topic relevant to their profession and practice. In some courses, assignments are assessed and graded solely on the basis of whether they meet publication standards and are suitable for submission for review and publication in a professional journal.

Each case should be judged on its own individual merits. My own assessment of whether an assignment, essay or a minor thesis contains material that is suitable for publication depends on my appraisal of:

- the subject of the essay/assignment/minor thesis and whether it stands to make a significant contribution of knowledge to the field
- how well the work has been written and whether it complies with the standards expected of writing that is published in professional journals and texts.

Contributions are useful and stand to make 'a significant contribution of knowledge to the field' when:

- they expand on or clarify what others have said
- they offer alternative perspectives
- they make connections with related subjects
- they make a material difference to the status quo
- the new or innovative dimension(s) of the work can be discerned and explained (Rankin 2001; Thomas 2000).

Students and academic or professional staff contemplating revising and submitting coursework essays and assignments for publication need to consider carefully the following questions:

1. Does my work stand to make a significant contribution of knowledge to the field and to the 'professional conversations' that are going on? In particular, does the work:
   • expand on or clarify what others have said
   • offer an alternative perspective to that which is already established in the field?
   • make a connection with other related subjects?
   • prompt a change in policy and/or practice?
   • exhibit the hallmarks of being new or innovative, and can these hallmarks be discerned and explained?
2. Does my work uphold the principles of a 'good' writing style (such as those discussed in Chapter 3) and comply with the standards expected of academic or professional writing?

All writers should, of course, ask these questions, not just novice student-writers. This is because, as Elizabeth Rankin (2001, p. 10) correctly advises:

As writers our first obligation is to think about what we are contributing to [professional] conversation— what new information, insight, theoretical perspective,

argument, application, approach, or deepened understanding we have to share with others in the field.

PREPARING CONFERENCE PAPERS FOR PUBLICATION

Many health professionals and academics prepare papers
for presentation at conferences and seminars with the
intention of revising them later for publication in a
professional journal. A question they often ask is: 'How
do I go about revising a conference paper for publication?' The short answer to this question is: *prepare the
paper as an article for publication in the first place* and *then*
present its key points to a conference audience, not the
other way round.

Writing a paper for presentation at a conference with
the *intention* of later revising it for publication is a *trap*.
Once a paper has been presented at a conference, it is more
likely to languish in a file 'waiting' for revision, than is a
paper that has been prepared adequately from the start for
submission to a journal and from which an author has
made a presentation. An audience can always read the finer
details of what you have written at another time. When
presenting a paper, focus on getting a message across: *speak
from the head, the heart and the soul.* Then refer the
audience to what you have written and where they can
locate it (either now or at some future point in time) so
that they might consider and digest the finer points.

If you do fall into the trap of 'presenting now, writing
later', the principles of converting an assignment into an
article or book chapter apply (see section earlier in this
chapter) as do the principles of scholarly writing and
writing well as discussed in Chapter 3.

MAKING REVISIONS

No work is complete until it has undergone some revision. Although a normal and necessary part of the writing process, making revisions is not necessarily an easy task. How well you deal with the task of revising your work—and how productive it is in terms of improving the overall quality of your work—will depend as much on your *attitude* toward it, as it does on your skill as a writer. Elizabeth Rankin's (2001) advice on this matter is unequivocal: *learn to like it!*

Revising a work is undertaken fundamentally for the purpose of *improving the work*, and involves rigorous editing that has as its focus:

- checking the manuscript for accuracy and clarity
- removing incorrect or unwanted matter
- selecting, rearranging or rejecting material included in the original draft
- altering or amending material to ensure 'fit' and compliance with the principles of style.

The main difficulty faced by writers when revising their work is deciding *what* to let go and then, *letting it go* (Rankin 2001, p. 82). Here the rule of 'natural selection' applies: *allow and retain only those ideas and material that are pertinent, necessary and 'best adapted' to the survival and success of the work.*

Arguably a greater challenge for writers is when they are required *by others* (often anonymous reviewers) to make major revisions and to redraft large sections of the work. This can be a frustrating and disheartening experience. If, however, the revisions stand to improve the work, then attend to the revisions with diligence and grace. If the revisions requested do not stand to improve the work and worse, may even undermine its integrity (as can sometimes happen), this is another matter entirely. Your best option in a situation like this is to not make the revisions requested and to write a carefully considered defence of why you have not made the changes requested. Depending on how your defence is received, respond accordingly.

Finally, there is the challenge of deciding *yourself* that major revisions are required. Provided this decision is not driven by a faulty appraisal of the merits and quality of your work, and feedback from others confirms and validates your own appraisal, simply sit down and undertake the revisions. As the King said to the White Rabbit in *Alice's Adventures in Wonderland*: 'Begin at the beginning and go on till you come to the end: then stop' (Carroll 1962, p. 154). Know, however, when to stop.

SPELLING, GRAMMAR AND OTHER STYLISTIC ISSUES

Many manuscripts 'fail' because the writer has not mastered the fundamentals of writing: *spelling, grammar* and *style*. Unless a writer has competence in these things it will not be possible to develop competence as a writer, let alone become a 'good' writer. If you feel that your skills in this area need development then you may need to consider undertaking a course (for example, at an adult learning centre such as a local Council for Adult Education) or undertaking some self-directed learning on the subject, such as by studying books and manuals on the topics of spelling, grammar and style. Examples of such works include:

- *Style Manual* (6th edition) published by John Wiley & Sons, 2002.
- *The Art of Styling Sentences: 20 patterns for success* (4th edition) by A. Longknife and K. Sullivan, 2002.
- *The Penguin Writer's Manual* by M. Manser, and S. Curtis, 2002.
- *Publication Manual* (5th edition), American Psychological Association, Washington DC, 2001.

Another issue requiring attention is that of writers not using the correct spelling, terminology, or the correct words in their work. Spelling and the use of dictionaries are discussed in 'Choose your words' carefully in Chapter 3. In the case of the latter, it is good practice to have a small dedicated table near your writing desk or computer for your dictionary. This will allow easy access to it for checking words and, in turn, will help you to cultivate the habit of checking words regularly. I have a dictionary sitting near my computer and when I am writing it is rarely closed. While writing this chapter I consulted the dictionary no less than 20 times. Some of the words I needed to check to make sure they were the most appropriate or spelled correctly were:

- troubleshooting
- salient
- writer's block (not found in the dictionary)

- procrastination
- character
- personality
- natural selection (as in evolution)
- nomenclature
- facetious.

A final word of warning about spelling: *Never* rely on a computer spell checker to check the spelling in any writing you prepare for publication. They are not fool-proof and you do not have full control over the quality of the dictionary the computer uses for this function.

Finally, there is the issue of poor style—both in the structure of the work and in the expression of its content. As the issues of style and structure have already been addressed in Chapters 3 and 5, I shall make just two comments:

- pay attention to the elements and principles of style
- pay attention to the principles of structure.

Writing that is not presented in a clear, direct, simple, coherent and engaging manner will simply not be read.

BACK-UP COPIES

There has been many a sad story involving writers who have 'lost' their work on account of their computer malfunctioning or being stolen. There is one remedy for this situation: *always keep back-up copies*—both computer disk and hard copies—and store these in separate locations. When closing a file on your computer always copy it to a floppy disk and always print out a hard copy before shutting down the computer. Keep these back-up copies in a safe place (for example, one at home and one at work and even one at a friend's place). This is especially important when you have prepared the final copy of a manuscript. There can be nothing so devastating to a writer than losing a recently completed rigorously edited final copy of a work.

LIFESTYLE AND FINDING A BALANCE

Upon becoming engrossed in a writing career it can be easy to lose sight of the outside world and to forget that you have other lives—as a partner, lover, friend, parent, sibling, co-worker, pet owner. My advice here is: do not lose sight of your other lives and remember *to have a life*. Your success as a writer will not mean very much if you—or those close to you—are not around to enjoy it.

Make sure that in addition to making time to write, you also make time to have fun and to sustain and nurture the important relationships in your life. The motivational writer John Kehoe (1998, p. 167) suggests, facetiously, that we should all try to have fun at least three times a day! In response to the question, How much time does it take to have fun?, he writes in a more serious tone:

> Sometimes just a few moments. You can have fun in almost any situation. When you are driving to work and enjoying a good song on the radio—that's fun. A joke shared with a fellow employee, a chapter read in a good novel, even a brisk walk in the sunshine or a workout at the gym can be fun.

As an academic or clinician, adding a writing schedule to your daily activities is likely to make your busy life even busier. It is vital therefore that every effort is made to achieve a balance between work and play. One way of doing this is to designate some 'sacred time' during each week for engaging in the things that are meaningful and which give rise to a sense of joy.

Include in your writing schedule a 'sacred time' slot each week and do not allow this time to be violated. Sacred time must be set aside each week to do such things as: spending time with loved ones; going for walks; cycling or horse riding; eating out at a favourite restaurant; watching a favourite television program; going to a movie; and just generally spending time doing the things that matter. There is no shame in taking time out; if there is a shame to be had, it is in the fact of *not* taking enough time out to attend to the things that really matter and which make life meaningful. To those who say that they cannot afford to take time out, my response is: *you cannot afford NOT to take time out*.

SUMMARY

All writers will encounter certain difficulties during the course of their writing careers. Many of these difficulties are normal and expected, and most can be resolved, such as by using the strategies discussed in this book.

Although writing (and the problems associated with it) can be very challenging, it can also be very rewarding. Most successful writers will concede that, despite the difficulties—despite the headaches the backaches and the soul aches—at the end of the day, it has all been worth it.

EXERCISES

1. Make a list of problems you have experienced or anticipate experiencing during the course of your writing career.
2. Outline how you dealt with the problems you experienced.
3. Outline a plan of how you propose to deal with a problem you anticipate you will experience in the future.

7 | PROMOTING YOUR WORK

'Writer's names are inextricably linked to their work. People buy a particular book, go to a movie or a play because they know that the author's professional reputation carries with it distinctive qualities with which they can identify. Getting your name known is as important for art as for mass-produced items.'

—Day (1993, p. 8)

'If you want to succeed you have to look to yourself.'
—Archer (1991, p. 40)

There is a cultural expectation in places like NZ, Australia and the UK that writer's will be appropriately self-effacing and modest about their writing accomplishments and will play down any praise that they may get. Susan Mitchell (2000, p. 99), for example, observed that when the Australian actor Geoffrey Rush won an Oscar award for best actor in the film *Shine*,

> . . . he went out of his way to prove that it really was no big deal and that fame would not change him. After the initial burst of world-wide publicity he did not splash his face across every newspaper and magazine in endless interviews and when he did make public utterances they were always suitably self-effacing.

Writers, especially academic writers, who breach the unwritten cultural expectation of 'keep your talents hidden under a bushel' risk not only being treated with suspicion, but also being criticised and ostracised by their colleagues (recall Susan Mitchell's experience of the 'Politics of Envy', referred to on page 84 of this book). For some reason, academics who are successful authors particularly fear 'being branded as populist by other academics' (Thomas 2000, p. 120), and in most instances do not—and prefer not—to see themselves as *writers* at all. On this latter point, the author bell hooks (1999, p. 37) notes with irony: 'All academics write but not all see themselves as writers'.

As I stated in Chapter 1 of this book, professional scholarship and publishing is an important issue and activity for the health professions. Given the importance of published work reaching a broad audience—particularly where the works in question could have an important influence on promoting the health and wellbeing of people and even saving lives—the cultural expectation to be 'appropriately self-effacing' (which, for academic writers, can mean *being silent*) it is not only absurd but may even be unethical. Indeed, there are many examples in history where professional jealousies and envy saw the marginalisation of important works that, had they been widely disseminated, promoted and accepted at the time, could have improved the wellbeing or saved the lives of thousands and even millions of people. To cite just three examples:

• had the reports by Drs Holmes and Semmelweiss, during the 1840s, on the cause and spread of puerperal sepsis been accepted by the medical profession at the time (they in fact ignored Semmelweiss's recommendations for 60 years), thousands of women could have been prevented from contracting the disease and dying or having total hysterectomies as a result (Nadelson and Notman 1978, p. 1716);

- had the articles on child abuse first published in the *British Medical Journal* in the 1860s not been ignored, the medical profession in common law countries could have made a major contribution to the prevention and treatment of child abuse *one hundred years* before it eventually did so (Johnstone 1999b, pp. 65–76, 91–9);

- had important early articles on the nature of the tubercule bacillus and possible means of penetrating its outer membrane to allow its effective treatment not got 'lost in the shuffle' or treated, as they were, with disbelief by sections of the medical profession, not only would a cure for tuberculosis have been found much earlier than it was but we may possibly even not be facing the new drug-resistant tuberculosis epidemic that we are today (Ryan 1992).

There is a place for 'appropriate' modesty and there is a place for 'good manners' in the way you go about discussing your achievements. Certainly, boasters can be irritating and you do not want to put people off *you* and hence *your work*. But there is no place for keeping quiet about a published work that could influence policy and practice in a manner that would improve significantly the lives and wellbeing of others who are vulnerable. I believe that not only is it acceptable for such work to be promoted, but it is morally imperative to do so.

There is no point publishing an important work only to have it sit gathering dust on some forgotten bookshelf in a library or office. Ignore the critics, promote your work and snatch the headlines. If you feel uncomfortable about this, think of the times your life or professional practice has been affected in positive ways by attending a conference, or reading a book or an article that someone has recommended to you, or which you first heard about on the radio or read about in a review. Think also of the times that people who have had their lives (personal and professional) shaken on account of 'not knowing' about a development and hence not being able to take corrective or curative action to improve the status quo.

There are three key ways in which your publications can be promoted appropriately and effectively, namely via:

- seminar and conference presentations
- listing them as educational references in tertiary education or professional practice development programs
- media publicity (both print and electronic).

SEMINAR AND CONFERENCE PRESENTATIONS

A useful and important way to promote your work is through seminar and conference presentations. Performance as a public speaker at seminar and conference venues is a good way to:

- get valuable feedback on your ideas (audiences are rarely slow or shy in voicing their opinions)
- enable your readers to gain access to you and to feel a sense of connection with a 'real' person and his or her work (ultimately it is your readers who are your greatest advertisement and you should look after them; being accessible is one way of showing them respect and 'looking after them')
- develop a professional network and facilitate the dissemination of the work.

In regard to the latter opportunity, Marele Day (1993, p. 76) contends:

Networking—using personal contacts—should not be underestimated or seen in a negative light. Commercial and professional dealings through personal relations has a long history. People feel more inclined to support a known rather than an unknown factor. Your willingness to know the people in your industry and to maintain contact with them is a measure of your commitment to that industry and your place in it.

When attending a seminar or conference as a presenter, it is entirely appropriate to:

- present the findings of your work in your paper
- network to foster the promotion of your work by others
- promote your work yourself (for example, by holding a book signing session).

UTILISATION OF SCHOLARSHIP IN EDUCATION AND PROFESSIONAL PRACTICE DEVELOPMENT

There is a curious reticence among many academics to list their own works as references in the educational and professional development programs they facilitate and teach. This situation is perhaps partially explained by the unwritten cultural rules of modesty and demands to play down one's achievements, discussed in the opening paragraphs to this chapter. Other possible reasons remain a matter for speculation. Regardless, it seems odd that an academic or professional writer who cares deeply about their work and who writes largely to influence change and to participate in the professional conversations that are occurring at the time, should choose not to share their work with students and colleagues at the forefront of practice.

Another problem is when colleagues refuse to list or recommend your works. I know of cases where an academic's publications have been listed as recommended reading for students and cited widely by colleagues *outside* of their teaching institutions yet are barely mentioned in the corridors where they work.

Students and colleagues *deserve* to have access to new publications in a timely manner *and* to the people who write them. Further, it is well recognised that students and participants at seminars and conferences prefer their facilitators, speakers and teachers to have a well-established professional reputation and to have international standing in their fields. Many educational institutions also now demand that academics demonstrate a critical link between their research, scholarship, teaching and professional practice, and how each has informed the other.

It is important to recognise that teaching and practice can be a valuable source of ideas for research and scholarship, and vice versa. It is not immodest or 'wrong' and indeed it is entirely appropriate to:

- list your publications, where relevant, as recommended reading in the educational programs that you teach or facilitate
- make your publications available to others such as by ordering them for or placing them on 'closed reserve' in a library
- recommend your work to others for educational and professional development purposes.

In addition, work to break the 'politics of envy' that may be operating in your workplace environment. Lead by example and praise the work of your colleagues by:

- commending and recommending their publications to others
- making reference to their publications in your own work
- including their publications in your recommended readings lists for students
- acknowledging the kudos their successful publications are bringing to your organisation and to those associated with it
- giving them positive feedback (everyone loves positive feedback!)

Former English Conservative prime minister, Sir Winston Churchill (1875–1965), achieved many things in this life. Describing the man and his achievements, a reporter once wrote of Winston Churchill, 'He is a modest man who has a good deal to be modest about' (*Chicago Sunday Tribune Magazine of Books*, 1954). The same can be said for successful authors whose work has a positive impact on the learning and practice of others.

MEDIA PUBLICITY

Undoubtedly one of the best means of attracting public attention to your work is the *media*. Most universities and health care agencies have a public relations department or unit that can assist and facilitate you in obtaining media attention to your work. These units can assist your publicity cause by working closely with you to formulate media releases, putting you in contact with journalists and arranging interviews with either radio or television broadcasters. The advantages of media publicity are that:

- it is free
- it will help spread knowledge of your work and its findings to a broader audience
- it brings kudos to your employing institution, your profession and to you
- it helps to further the reputation of your department/university/health care agency as a centre of excellence
- it demonstrates the impact of your work (it has been deemed worthy of notice).

There are, however, also a number of disadvantages in getting your work publicised in the media. These include:

- the reports may not come out when you want them to
- the reports may not appear where you want them to (they may, for example, appear on page 60 of a newspaper instead of page 3, or better still, page 1; or they may appear only in regional papers, not in the newspapers that enjoy mass circulation)
- the reports may not be accurate and may contain misleading information or quote you incorrectly
- journalists and broadcasters may only be able to contact you for comment out of hours or during highly inconvenient times, such as very early in the morning or extremely late at night (I have done interviews at 5 a.m. and midnight, on the way to the airport and in the middle of dinner)
- the publicity you get may be 'bad'
- your privacy may be intruded upon by a public whose interest has been aroused in your work (expect to get unsolicited phone calls and letters—both good and bad).

To ensure that you get the best out of media publicity of your work, ensure that you:

- *have* a media strategy
- foster a good relationship with the team in your university's or health care agency's public relations department/unit (keep them informed, give them timely notice of a pending story, treat them with courtesy and respect, respond quickly to their requests for information and comment)

- foster a good relationship with sympathetic journalists and broadcasters (be available and accessible, respond quickly to their calls, ensure they are briefed well about your work and in a timely manner, always be courteous and professional in your dealings with them, give them 'first option' on doing an exclusive report)
- keep a list and the contact details of possible media outlets relevant to your field
- have something interesting to publicise
- be clear about the message you want to get across in the media
- undergo media training (this can be very helpful if you are likely to be interviewed by radio or television journalists and broadcasters)(see also Baverstock 2002).

SUMMARY

It is important that once a work is published every effort is made to ensure that it becomes known to its potential readers. In professional and academic circles often the best way to promote a published work is via professional seminars and conferences, and through the recommended readings of staff development or formal education courses.

Although some health professionals and academic writers are reluctant to publicise their work, obtaining publicity is a normal and necessary part of the writing process and, in many instances, may even be a moral imperative. It is generally accepted that the writing process is complete once a manuscript has been *published*. I would suggest, however, that the writing process is never complete until the work has been published, promoted and *publicised*.

EXERCISES

1. Obtain the names and contact details of the staff working in the public relations or media unit in your employing institution.
2. Clarify the process for engaging their assistance when seeking publicity for your work
3. Undertake a short media training course.

8 | AUTHOR RIGHTS AND RESPONSIBILITIES

'Without academic freedom, there is no integrity in academe. And when academic integrity is breached in any way, the result is the betrayal of academic freedom.'
—Sheinin (1993, p. 234)

'Accountability in the academy comes not from statistics collected for outputs and outcomes, but from the hard scrutiny of open publication and academic debate.'
—McCalman (2000, p. 17)

Writing and publishing never occur in a moral or legal vacuum and are never free of moral or legal risks. It is important, therefore, that you have some knowledge and understanding of your rights, responsibilities and duties as a writer and author, and how you might be assisted to exercise these. Furthermore, it is important to understand that ethical and legal issues can arise during and after, and can affect 'all stages of the writing process: researching, interviewing, quoting from other material and ownership of your work' (Maskell and Perry 1999, p. 25).

ACADEMIC FREEDOM

A key issue facing writers who work in the tertiary education sector and, more recently, who work in research-oriented health care service organisations, is that of *academic freedom*. Regrettably, in recent times the notion of academic freedom has become misunderstood and sometimes perverted to serve the vested interests of an elite few. For example, some tertiary education union representatives reportedly believe that academic freedom means the freedom of individual academics to work 'when and where they please' without having to let others (such as their managers and colleagues) know where they can be contacted if required urgently during usual weekday working hours (Madden 2001, p. 26). This view is, however, at odds with the original purpose of academic freedom, and its counterpart *academic integrity*, which I'll discuss in the next section of this chapter.

The notion of academic freedom dates back to the sixth century and the 'democratic philosophy and practice of men and women who came together as teachers and scholars in the Benedictine monasteries . . . to share learning and knowledge in a common collective' (Sheinin 1993, p. 233). For an 800-year period after this time, however, the religious fathers of the day and their followers overturned the ideals, processes and practice of academic freedom and its democratic underpinnings. Notable among these were the followers of the Italian theologian, St Thomas Aquinas (1225–74), who imposed the authoritarian and hierarchal structure of the Church of Rome on universities—a structure that was replicated in universities not only across Europe, but across the world, including those found in the major cities and nation states of the Middle East, South Asia, the continent of Africa and the Americas (both north and south) and which persist to this day (Sheinin 1993, p. 233).

Major casualties of the thirteenth century 'university restructuring' were women. In accordance with papal decree, women were specifically excluded from the academy and thereby obstructed from pursuing scholarly activities. It was not until the Reformation in the sixteenth century that academic freedom and its demo-cratic ideals regained their currency and which remains a cornerstone of professorial appointment to this day. Although it has been variously interpreted and, at times, grossly misinterpreted for questionable purposes, there is nevertheless a consensus that the notion of academic freedom fundamentally embraces the rights (and duties) of those in the academy to:

> . . . speak their thoughts, their beliefs, and their sen-timents in full and open freedom in the secure sense that, should these not always be in accord with those spoken by the rest of society, the individual and collec-tive status of those who express them, as members of the guild of teachers and scholars of the university, will in no way be threatened (Sheinin 1993, p. 235).

For the purposes of this discussion, the term academic freedom, as it relates to writing and publication in health care, is taken to mean the freedom of health professionals (including clinicians, academics and their students) to be independent in their intellectual thinking, action and personality and to 'hold opinions, especially unorthodox opinions, and to advocate them openly and without fear of reprisal' (Arblaster 1974, p. 14). It encompasses freedom:

- of thought
- of inquiry
- of speech
- of expression
- from the threat and practice of physical and psychological violence
- from oppression and suppression
- from exclusion, marginalisation and ostracism (Sheinin 1993, pp. 235–6).

This view rests on the assumption that an important and fundamental social function of the modern academy is to be: 'critical, questioning, experimental and innovatory' (Arblaster 1974, p. 22), and that people in the academy not only have a *right* to speak out but a fundamental moral *duty* to do so—especially in political contexts where the freedom to speak and act is under threat. As the intellectual Edward Said (1994) persuasively argues, the fundamental task of the intellectual is to 'rock the boat' by straying outside the margins of accepted paradigms and, assuming a principled stance, confronting the difficult. In his essay on *Speaking Truth to Power*, Said (1994, p. 75) writes:

> Speaking truth to power is no Panglossian [all inclusive, bright and glossy] idealism: it is carefully weighing the alternatives, picking the right one, and then intelligently representing it where it can do the most good and cause the right change.

In recent times, the academic freedom of writers has been placed increasingly under threat, with universities being accused publicly around the world of 'stifling debate' and putting pressure on academics to comply with the status quo (James 1999; McCalman 2000; McPhee 2002; Sheinin 1993). In the United States, for example, academics have been dismissed from their jobs for speaking out against government policy following the 2001 September 11 terrorist attack on the twin towers in New York. Criticising this assault on academic freedom, one commentator is reported as stating, 'At a moment such as this we must make sure that all informed voices, especially those that are critical and dissenting, are heard' (Major 2001, p. 13). It was reported that students were among those 'calling for action against academics who question the US Government's actions' (Major 2001, p. 13).

Academic freedom in writing and publishing is concerned with challenging the status quo and with producing work that is:

- questioning
- critical
- innovative
- experimental.

It is also concerned with 'pricking our collective conscience' (McPhee 2002, p. 13).

When expressing academic freedom, the means to achieving those ends must always be *moral*, that is, be done for the *right* reasons, in the *right* way and for the *right* outcome. In other words, academic freedom must be expressed with, and constrained by, *academic integrity*.

ETHICAL CONSIDERATIONS

As I mentioned in the opening paragraph to this chapter, writing and publishing never occur in a moral vacuum and are never free of moral risks. Despite this, curiously little has been written on the subject of *writing ethics* or *author ethics*. Where references have been made to the ethical dimensions of writing and publishing these have tended to be brief and of a nature simply reminding authors to *be ethical* and to consult and uphold relevant professional codes of practice during the course of their work (for example, journalists are advised to consult their local Journalists' Association *Code of Ethics*).

Professional and academic writing and publication can be an intensely political act. This is especially so in contexts where the writing aims to challenge the status quo (such as an established but questionable policy, practice or some other convention) and to *do something about it*, not merely be a passive observer of what is going on.

Writing can have the power to *honour* (give glory to), *liberate* (make free) and *integrate* (bring together) people and/or their ideas. A poignant example of this can be found in the influential works written by the Brazilian educationalist Paulo Freire, especially his *Pedagogy of the Oppressed* (which has sold over 500 000 copies world wide) and *Cultural Action for Freedom*—both first published in 1970. Freire's early work helped to empower countless impoverished and illiterate people in Brazil, the consequences of which were so threatening to the authorities of the day that Freire was forced into exile for 20 years.

Freire's works continue to be influential around the world over thirty years after first being published—particularly in countries seeking to unite, empower and make free indigenous peoples whose cultures and lives have been torn apart by the legacies of colonialism. His ideas have been and continue to be applied by a wide range of people, including psychologists, social workers, counsellors, theologians and educationalists, working in hospitals, prisons, schools, adult education programs and universities (Roberts 1999). When *Pedagogy of the Oppressed* was first published in an English language edition it was regarded not just as an accomplishment but as a *prophet event*, and one that continues to have a fundamental impact in countries whose peoples are burdened by economic, social and political oppression.

Unfortunately, writing also has the power to *dishonour* (treat with disrespect), *imprison* (confine) and *corrupt* (literally, to break things to pieces). A sobering example of this can be found in the case notes, daily reports and professional publications of Nazi doctors and allied health professionals, including eugenicists, psychiatrists and nurses (Caplan 1992; Lifton 1986; McFarland-Icke 1999). These works played a vital role in supporting and sustaining the daily regimes and routines of Hitler's medicalised killing programs that, between 1939–45, resulted in over 100 000 patients with mental or physical disabilities being killed (McFarland-Icke 1999). It is important (and devastating) to note that the publications of the scientific disciplines (especially the biomedical disciplines)—by advancing 'scientific racism'—also enabled the most vicious forms of anti-Semitism to emerge and flourish during this period by bestowing on them both scientific legitimacy and intellectual respectability (Lifton 1986, p. 17). Equally troubling is that the Nazi doctors and eugenicists who were at the forefront of influencing social and public health policy at the time were not unique in their views; racial eugenics enjoyed passionate support in the United States of American and the United Kingdom as well—and long before the Nazis came to power (Lifton 1986, p.23). What is unique, however, is the way in which these disciplines supported and advanced the use of medical metaphor in and successfully blended it with 'concrete biomedical ideology in the Nazi sequence from coercive sterilisation to direct medical killing to the death camps' (Lifton 1986, p. 16).

These and other historical examples demonstrate that writers need to be ever mindful that writing and its publication has the power to challenge and change the status quo. This power, however, can be negative as well as positive, and can have harmful as well as beneficial outcomes. For this reason, writers must remain vigilant and ensure that their writing is morally responsible, and the power it exerts morally justified.

When you write, remember always that what you put into print could have a significant impact on the lives and wellbeing of others. It is the capacity to affect significantly the moral interest of others that most imposes on the writer a moral duty to exercise care in his or her work and to uphold the most stringent moral standards both when:

- determining the object or purpose of their writing
- when engaging in the process of writing itself.

When developing your writing career and engaging in the writing process it is imperative that you uphold the agreed ethical and professional conduct standards of your profession. Many of these commonly accepted standards are as relevant to the purposes and processes of professional and academic writing as they are for guiding professional practice. Over and above this, however, there is also a fundamental ethical standard that applies to writers (and to editors and publishers), namely, the virtue of *integrity*.

Integrity at its most basic is adherence to moral principles. It is, however, also much more than this: it is adherence to the quality and practice of *moral excellence* and to exhibiting conduct that is of an *exceptionally high standard*—that is, a standard that is generally higher than that which would otherwise be expected of others not engaged in a professional activity. It is conduct that is 'unimpaired' and sound in every way.

Arguably, the most important moral qualities a writer can exhibit when engaged in the writing process derive from the system and theory of ethics called *virtue ethics* and encompass the four interrelating cardinal virtues of: prudence, justice, fortitude and temperance. Consider the following:

Prudence

To be prudent is to exercise good judgement, to be discreet and cautious in managing one's activities, and to be practical and careful in providing for the future.

During all phases of the writing process, writers must exercise good judgement and be careful, cautious and discrete in their writing, in deciding the purpose of their writing, in the means they use for obtaining material to inform their writing and in getting their work published. Writers also need to be practical and manage the writing process to ensure their future success as writers: *what and how you write now could have an important bearing on what, if and when you will write in the future.*

When engaged in the writing process, ensure that you uphold the following 'golden rules' of author conduct:

- *Authenticity*—ensure that your work builds on and advances a genuine, reliable and accurate representation of 'the facts' or issues at hand; do not falsify data or exaggerate their significance; avoid taking a 'straw man' position, that is, inventing a problem that does not exist and addressing it in preference to the real issues or arguments held by others.
- *Honesty*—ensure that your writing is genuine, sincere, just and authentic; do not deliberately mislead your readers, editors or publishers; do not plagiarise the work of others; take all challenges to your work seriously and respond to them with tolerance, compassion, intelligence and in an open and informed manner; when in doubt seek advice.
- *Beneficence*—write primarily for the purposes of contributing beneficial knowledge to the field, of demonstrating public accountability and improving the status quo, rather than for self-aggrandisement; remember that writing is a social service—its principal

aim is to serve the public interest (that is, the protection of the public and the public's moral goods/benefits, concerns or interests) and to improve the status quo, not to serve yourself.

Justice

Justice refers to fairness and to the equal distribution of benefits and burdens. During the writing process, writers must ensure that they *deal fairly* with others (their co-authors, editors, publishers, managers, colleagues, other subjects/participants) and must *represent fairly* the issues, ideas and entities (people, groups, communities, organ-isations, institutions, nations) they may be writing about. A failure to be just could have harmful and otherwise preventable moral consequences to innocent others, who could be unjustly damaged and even destroyed by the views, revelations and arguments presented in a writer's publications. A failure to be just could also harm the writer: their professional reputation and career as a writer could be damaged irreparably.

When engaged in the writing process, ensure that you uphold the principles of:

*   *Respect*—treat the people, issues and competing ideas that you are working with in a manner that is honest, authentic, respectful, credible and free of unwarranted biases and prejudices (noting here that sometimes justice requires 'positive discrimination', that is, treating entities *unequally* so that the least well off will gain access to an equal share of the benefits that only the most well off enjoy and enjoy exclusively).

- *Privacy and informed consent*—respect your collaborators' prima facie right to privacy and the right to give an informed consent for the use of any personal or private material that you may wish to quote in your work. (It is generally accepted that people have a prima facie moral right to have control over information about themselves and about who should have access to it and for what purposes—particularly where the information is of a nature that could harm significantly their moral interests; provided there exist no strong moral reasons to override these rights, you have an obligation to respect them.)

- *Distributive justice*—respect the conventions of submitting work for publication; ensure only those who make a significant contribution to a work (including yourself) are cited as authors to the work (do not 'free ride' on the work of others and do not allow others to free ride on your work); do not submit the same article to more than one journal at a time (this may unfairly use a journal's limited peer-review and editorial resources and compromise its publishing program in the event that an article accepted for publication is subsequently withdrawn); declare any conflict of interest (particularly when participating in a peer-review process) since this will help to ensure that there is not an unfair distribution of benefits and burdens as can happen when authors have their manuscripts unfairly rejected by a reviewer who is an open competitor with their work and, conversely, unfairly accepted by a reviewer who is a champion and advocate of their work.

Fortitude

To have fortitude is to have strength and firmness of mind. A distinguishing characteristic and virtue of a good writer is *intellectual rigour*. Intellectual rigour relates to the capacity of a writer to understand, think and reason in a strictly disciplined, credible, undistracted and trustworthy way.

Another distinguishing feature of a good writer is *credibility*. The credibility of a writer rests not only on his or her experience, track record, standing in the field and professionalism, but also on his or her commitment to the writing process—seeing the project through to the end, contributing to professional conversations, being publicly accountable, being prepared to 'stand up and be counted', being accessible to readers and constituents, and to producing work that is believable and which has practical application to solving real world problems.

When engaged in the writing process, uphold the principles of:

- *Competence*—have the appropriate skills, knowledge and capability to write well; do not undertake projects that are beyond your ability and which may leave your editors, publishers and readers feeling as though they have been 'cheated' and let down.
- *Conscientiousness*—be diligent and take painstaking care in researching material for your work and in writing your manuscripts (whether commentaries, opinion pieces, journal articles, book chapters, books or reports).
- *Conscience*—have a strong and conscientious sense of 'right' and 'wrong' when thinking about and doing

your work; faithfully represent (that is, do not deliberately misinterpret or misrepresent) the views and ideas of others; give appropriate acknowledgement to the work of others when you use it to inform your own work (do not steal their ideas and claim them as your own); do not misrepresent, falsify or exaggerate the importance of your own work; do not falsify the methods or results of your research; do not obstruct the career development and writing aspirations of others out of fear and envy; do not claim or allow others to claim authorship that is not authentic.

- *Courage*—deal with and act appropriately and effectively in the face of fear, pain, threat or danger; have the 'courage of your convictions'—act in accordance with your moral values and beliefs, and be willing to 'take a stand', particularly when doing so could prevent otherwise avoidable and foreseeable harms from occurring or promotes a benefit that would otherwise not be promoted if you did not take a stand; when vulnerable, seek support; if you make a mistake, admit it and apologise.

- *Commitment*—fulfil your obligations and promises even when doing so might sometimes involve curtailing your own interests; keep to the word limit, meet your deadlines, keep to the point; respect and honour the agreements you have entered into, provided this does not require you to breach other important moral standards.

Temperance

To act with temperance is to act with moderation and restraint. It is important that writers control their passions both when dealing with their constituents and when writing. Emotional outbursts and other behaviour that exceeds what is generally regarded as being socially acceptable will serve neither the author nor his or her work in either the immediate or long term. People may not remember what someone did on a particular occasion, but they will often remember how well or badly he or she responded.

Temperance should also be exercised in the *act* of writing. This is not to say that writing should be passionless and without life. To the contrary, as discussed in Chapter 5 of this book, writing that is written from the heart, the soul as well as the head can be inspiring and very successful in motivating people to act. It is quite a different matter, however, when writing is obsessive, overzealous, fanatical or even tyrannical in nature, the consequences of which can be dire. An important example of the kind of disastrous consequences that can occur as a result of the catalytic influences of an intemperate publication can be found in the case of Adolf Hitler's fanatical and influential work *Mein Kampf* in which Hitler expresses his views on the superiority of the Aryan race and the inferiority of the Jews.

When dealing with your constituents and when writing, ensure you uphold the interrelated and mutually constraining bioethical principles of:

- *Autonomy*—which prescribes that people should always be respected as self-determining choosers and should be respected as ends in themselves and not as the means to the ends of others; ensure that you treat your stakeholders with respect and do not use them as a means to achieving your writing goals.

- *Beneficence*—which prescribes and permits 'doing good'; ensure that your writing program and the processes for carrying it out are focused on achieving some specific morally benevolent ends such as the promotion of the interests of vulnerable people, or improving policy and practice for the benefit of all.

- *Nonmaleficence*—which prohibits decisions and actions that cause harm to others (it also prescribes the active prevention of harm where this can be done without sacrificing other important moral interests); ensure that your writing program and the processes for carrying it out will not cause otherwise avoidable harm to others and is focused, where relevant, on the prevention of harm.

- *Justice*—which prescribes actions that are fair, and which ensure an equal distribution of benefits and burdens; ensure that your writing program and the processes for carrying it out are fair and will not result in an unequal distribution of benefits and burdens to stake-holders (for an in-depth discussion of these principles see Beauchamp and Childress 2001).

Good writing is not merely technically correct or stylistically expert, it is also *morally excellent* in that it serves a morally worthy purpose (a moral end) *and* uses moral processes in achieving its intended purpose (a moral means to an end). Writers who ignore or violate the principles and prescriptions of ethical writing risk harming and bringing into disrepute themselves, their profession and their employer organisations.

LEGAL CONSIDERATIONS

Through all stages of the writing process, writers must remain vigilant in regard to the legal dimensions of writing and publishing. They need to make sure they are well informed about their legal rights and responsibilities and, in the event of a dispute, know where to go to get legal assistance either in the form of advice, mediation or court action.

Publishing law (particularly in the areas of copyright and libel) is an extremely complex and highly specialised area. Although an adequate explanation about all the legal issues relevant to writing and publishing is beyond the scope of this present work, it is worth highlighting a number of general points about:

- the publishing contract and obtaining legal advice
- copyright
- defamation.

The publishing contract

All book publishers and many (although not all) professional journals will issue you with a contract prior to commencing or, in the case of journals, publishing a work. When issued with such a contract it is not only highly advisable but imperative to seek legal advice from a lawyer conversant with publishing law before signing it. Just as you would not sign a contract for building or buying a house without getting legal advice, likewise you should not sign a contract for writing a book, book chapter or publishing a journal article without getting legal advice. General legal advice on a publishing contract for authors in Australia, the UK and New Zealand respectively can be obtained from:

- Australian Society of Authors (which offers a subsidised contract advice service for members; for further information visit the ASA website at <http://www.asauthors.org> and look up 'Contracts')
- The UK Society of Authors (which offers contract advice for members as well as legal representation when pursuing legal actions for breach of contract, copyright infringement and other publishing-related issues; for further information visit the Society of Authors website at <www.societyofauthors.org>)
- The New Zealand Society of Authors (for further information visit the NZ Society of Authors website at: <www.arachna.co.nz/nzsa>)
- Lawyers in private practice specialising in publishing and copyright law (since legal fees can be expensive, ensure you receive a quote before engaging a lawyer).
- Specialised legal advice on copyright issues may also be obtained without charge from the Australian Copyright Council (provided the issue on which you are seeking advice is *not* addressed in an Australian Copyright Council information sheet—available at <http://www.copyright.org.au/page3.htm>—and is not a matter of dispute before a court or of other legal proceedings). In the UK, advice can be obtained from the Copyright Licensing Agency (CLA) Ltd; (for further information visit the CLA website at <www.cla.co.uk>) and in New Zealand advice can be obtained from either the Copyright Council of New Zealand <www.copyright.org.nz> or Copyright Licensing Ltd <www.copyright.co.nz>. The issue of copyright is discussed in more detail below.

Most reputable publishers have 'standard' contracts. These contracts do not contain any 'tricks' but they do not necessarily represent the author's interests either. There is always room to negotiate the provisions contained in a standard contract to reflect your particular interests and project. Reputable publishers have an interest in securing and retaining a good author and, provided your requested amendments are not unreasonable, agreement on changes can usually be reached.

When you receive a contract from a publisher there are four golden rules:

- read it VERY CAREFULLY and identify any provisions within it that you find unsatisfactory
- make sure that it protects both your *pecuniary interests* as well as your *moral rights*
- DO NOT SIGN THE CONTRACT until you have *read it thoroughly*, have *received legal advice* and then *reached an agreement with the publisher* to amend any provisions you find unsatisfactory
- ensure you return the contract in a timely manner (if, because of waiting on legal advice or some other reason, you cannot meet the timeline specified by the publisher for returning the signed contract, formally request an extension to the timeline).

Copyright

A critical issue of mutual interest to authors, editors and publishers alike, and which is dealt with systematically in all publishing contracts, is the issue of *copyright*. Copyright refers to 'the exclusive right to reproduce or authorise others to reproduce artistic, dramatic, literary, or musical works' (*A Concise Dictionary of Law* 1990). Copyrights extend to sound broadcasting, computer works, film and live performances. Changes in Australian law that came into effect on 21 December 2000 (under the *Copyright Amendment (Moral Rights) Act 2000*) have extended copyright provisions to include 'moral rights' for creators. According to the Australian Copyright Council (2002a, pp. 1–2), under these provisions the creator of a work has the right to:

- be attributed as the creator of the work
- take action if his or her work is falsely attributed as being the work of someone else
- take action if his or her work is distorted or treated in a way that is prejudicial to his or her reputation (see also Australian Copyright Council 2001a).

The British *Copyright, Designs and Patents Act 1988* similarly provides for the protection of certain 'moral rights' in a work (Michaels 2003, p. 637).

In Australia, copyright provisions are contained in the commonwealth *Copyright Act 1968* and determined by the courts. In the UK, copyright provisions are contained in the *Copyright, Designs & Patents Act 1988*, that replaced the *Copyright Act 1956*, which in turn replaced the *Copyright Act 1911* (Michaels 2003). According to Michaels (2003, p. 629) 'all three Acts are still relevant to copyright today' in the UK.

Contrary to what some authors believe, provided a work is a creator's 'own' and not copied from someone else's work, copyright in the work is *automatic* and it is not essential therefore for a work to carry the © symbol (Australian Copyright Council 2002a; Legat 2003b). Inclusion of the sign may, however, 'act as a warning and help to stop another writer from plagiarising it' (Legat 2003b, p. 628).

Depending on the nature of the work, copyright in Australia usually lasts for the length of the author's life plus 50 years from the end of the year in which he or she died. In the UK, duration of copyright has been extended to 70 years from the end of the calendar year in which the author dies (Michaels 2003, p. 632).

Retaining, licensing and assigning copyright

At the heart of the copyright issue for authors is whether to and how to:

- retain exclusive copyright in their works
- 'lend' (license) the copyright in their works to others while retaining some rights to deal with the work
- 'sell' (assign) the copyright in their works to others and transfer all rights to the new owner.

The principle means by which copyrights in a work are distributed is via the legal contract (other means can include a written agreement, for example, as in the case of collaborating authors). When assigning or licensing their copyrights to a publisher, an author or creator of a work effectively relinquishes their otherwise exclusive rights to:

- publish the work for the first time
- publish the work using any form of technology (for example: computers, the Internet, audio recordings)

- reproduce the work (for example: by photocopying or photographing it, or scanning it onto a computer)
- perform the work in public
- make a translation or adaptation of the work (Australian Copyright Council 2001b, p. 1; see also Michaels 2003).

Most publishers insist on authors *assigning* their copyrights to them. Author groups, for example the ASA and the UK-based Society of Authors, however, generally advise authors only to *license* their works (Dunn 1999). This is because once the copyright in a work has been assigned an author generally loses all the above entitlements, or, at least, may have them severely limited. Likewise in the case of copyright being licensed, although to a lesser degree. In either case, it is critical that the conditions under which any or all of the rights might be restricted are *clearly specified* in the contract. For example, an author may assign all rights to a publisher, yet retain the right, on the condition of agreeing to give 'advice' to the publisher, to speak publicly about the work—including reciting excerpts from it—for the purposes of promoting and publicising it.

When negotiating a contract seek legal advice on the options you may have to limit the rights you are licensing or assigning to a publisher such as by specifying:

- the intended use of the work
- the circumstances under which further negotiation must be entered into (such as for a proposed electronic version or 'e-publication' of the work)

- the period of time for which use is granted (in any event, most book contracts have a sunset clause whereby all rights in a work revert back to the author in the event of the work going out of print or the publisher terminating the contract)
- territory where the work can be published (for example, the publisher should make clear what their intentions are of reproducing translations of the work for sale in overseas markets)
- other imposed conditions (for example, specifying that your name must appear on the cover, that the work cannot be used until consultancy fees have been paid, etc.)(see also Australian Copyright Council 2001b, p. 2; and the discussion on 'British copyright law' and 'US copyright law' in *Writers' & Artists' Yearbook 2003*, pp. 629–638, 644–652).

Copyright permission

Owners of copyright have the exclusive right to use copyright work in a variety of ways. This means that 'anyone who wants to use copyright material in any of these ways needs the copyright owner's permission' (Australian Copyright Council 2002a, p. 3 and Michaels 2003). Here, the demand to obtain permission to use copyright material (which, in essence, is a kind of 'property') is much like having to get permission to walk across someone else's land or enter someone else's property for some purpose.

Failure to obtain permission to use copyright material is normally regarded as an infringement of copyright and may be actionable in law unless copying falls under the 'fair-dealing' provisions as set out respectively in the *Australian Copyright Act 1968* and the UK *Copyright Designs & Patents Act 1988.* Section 41 of the *Australian Copyright Act* states that:

> A fair dealing with a literary, dramatic, musical or artistic work, or with an adaptation of a literary, dramatic or musical work, does not constitute an infringement of copyright in the work if it is for the purpose of criticism or review, whether of that work or of another, and a sufficient acknowledgement of the work is made.

The UK *Act* carries similar provisions at ss. 32–36 and elsewhere (Michaels 2003, pp. 634–636). What this means is that, under the fair dealing provisions, writers may quote other writers' work without having to seek permission *provided*:

- the material quoted is for 'the purpose of criticism or review'
- that 'sufficient acknowledgement' is made
- that the percentage of the material used is 'not substantial'.

In professional and academic writing the first two conditions can be readily satisfied. The latter condition, however, is not so easy to determine since the notion of 'substantial' is not defined in the respective *Copyright Acts* and is left to the discretion of the courts to decide on a case-by-case basis. In deciding what constitutes 'substantial', however, the courts will take into consideration not just the percentage or quantity of a work quoted or reproduced, but its *quality*. For example, a quote might be brief or a diagram small, but nevertheless be regarded as substantial on account of its originality.

In regard to ascertaining whether a quotation has infringed copyright, the Australian Copyright Council (2001c, p. 3) explains:

> Reproducing or communicating 10% of a work may be permissible for the purposes of research or study. Generally though, there is no standard percentage or proportion of a work or number of words than can be used without infringing copyright. In every case it is a question of whether an important, rather than a large, part of the work has been reproduced. Clearly, the number of words or proportion of a work which constitutes an important part will differ in every case.

In the UK, the *Copyright, Designs and Patents Act of 1988* permits up to '400 words of prose in a single extract from a copyright work, or a series of extracts of up to 300 words each, totalling no more than 800 words, or up to 40 lines of poetry, which must not be more than 25% of the poem', for the purposes of criticism or review (Legat 2003b, p. 627). Even in the case of these very specific provisions, however, deciding whether copyright has been upheld or infringed will require a case-by-case assessment.

Some clarification on how to assess whether dealing is 'fair' is provided by the English Justice, Lord Denning MR. In *Hubbard v. Vosper* (1972, p. 1027 [f–g]), Lord Denning took the position:

You must consider first the number and extent of quotations and extracts. Are they altogether too many and too long to be fair? Then you must consider the use made of them. If they are used as a basis for comment, criticism or review, that may be a fair dealing. If they are used to convey the same information as the author, but for a rival purpose, that may be unfair. Next, you must consider the proportions. To take long extracts and attach short comments may be unfair. But short extracts and long comments may be fair. Other considerations may come to mind also. But, after all is said and done, it must be a matter of impression.

It is generally accepted within Australia that up to 250 consecutive words is a reasonable limit for a 'fair dealing' quote, and up to 700 words of quotation *in total* is also acceptable 'for research or reviewing purposes without obtaining permission' (Dunn 1999, p. 161). In the UK, as just clarified, up to 400 consecutive words may be quoted, and up to 800 words of quotation *in total* may be used for research and review purposes without permission (Legat 2003b; Michaels 2003). If in doubt, seek advice from either your editor or publisher. Sometimes deciding whether you need to obtain copyright permission is analogous to deciding whether you should have insurance: *it is probably better to have it and not need it, than to not have it and need it.*

Legat (2003b) further advises UK authors: 'If you do not get a reply when you ask for permission to quote, insert a notice in your work saying that you have tried without success to contact the copyright owner, and would be pleased to hear from him or her so that the matter could be cleared up' (p. 627). He also advises authors to keep copies of all the releveant correspondence that was generated in your attempts to contact the copyright owners.

When quoting copyright material in your work, ensure that you:

- give due and proper acknowledgement to the copyright holder
- do not falsely attribute the work as being the work of someone else (including your own)
- do not distort or treat the material in a way that is prejudicial to the author's reputation
- obtain copyright permission to use quotes that are 'substantial' (either in quantity or quality)(Australian Copyright Council, 2001a, 2001c, 2002a; Legat 2003b; Michaels 2003)

Disputes about copyright

Sometimes there may be a dispute over who, in fact, holds copyright in a work. There are three ways of dealing with this situation:

- anticipate that it may occur and take appropriate steps to prevent it
- seek to have the matter resolved by mediation
- seek legal redress in a court of law.

When submitting manuscripts for publication get the manuscript post-stamped and send it by registered post to the publisher; at the same time, mail a copy of your manuscript to yourself with the same post-stamp on it. Leave the envelope sealed until the manuscript is formally accepted. This will stand as material evidence of the date and origin of a manuscript should your authorship of a work become the subject of a dispute (Dunn 1999, p. 155).

In the case of collaborative or commissioned works, ensure that an author agreement is in place in which the intellectual copyright entitlements of all co-participating entities have been clarified.

If there is a dispute about copyright, seek first to resolve the matter with the contesting parties either personally or, if that fails, by using a formal mediation service, such as the Arts Law Centre of Australia mediation service or the professional services that are provided to members by the UK-based Society of Authors. In the event that mediation is unsuccessful, you may have no choice (depending on the seriousness of the dispute and what is at issue) but to take the matter to court for resolution. If the matter does go to court, it will be necessary to provide material evidence supporting your copyright claims. Evidence may include, but not be limited to:

- oral evidence by the author
- evidence of witnesses (for example, those who may have directly observed the author working on a manuscript)
- drafts of work
- correspondence relating to the work

- the mail registration receipt and unsealed post-stamped manuscript and envelope referred to earlier (see also Australian Copyright Council 2002a, under subheading: 'How do I prove that I am the copyright owner if there is no system of registration').

Contractual obligations

All standard publishing contracts contain clauses and provisions covering copyright issues. These are commonly situated under subheadings, such as:

- Copyright, or Rights
- Auxiliary Material, Permissions and Index, or Delivery of Work and Ancillary Materials
- Commissioned Material
- Warranties.

Included under these clauses are the following worded provisions requiring the author to, among other things, confirm that the:

- Author grants the Publishers, for the legal period of copyright, the right and license to publish the work
- the work is an original work and does not infringe any existing copyright or any other right
- the Author has the full power and authority to enter into the Agreement and to grant the rights they consent to grant in the contract.

Defamation

To defame someone is to injure his or her good name and reputation in the eyes of reasonable members of the community and to cause reasonably minded people to avoid, ridicule or shun them (*A Concise Dictionary of Law* 1990; *Style Manual* 1994, 12.27; Watterson 1995a; Whitaker 2003).

A writer can defame a person by publishing material that is damaging to their reputation or good standing and can be sued accordingly for compensation for the injury and harm caused to that person's reputation (Maskell and Perry 1999, p. 25). Significantly, the majority of reported defamation cases in Australia and the UK have been against the media and have involved plaintiffs such as politicians, professionals, public officials and businessmen 'whose career or prosperity' have depended on their public reputations (Watterson 1995a, p. 10 Barendt et al. 1997).

Writers need to be aware that a person can be defamed not only when they are identified by name (*Style Manual* 1994, 12.28) but also if they are identified by nicknames or by innuendo (Watterson 1995a, p. 24 Whitaker 2003, p. 654). In Australia unintentional defamation of a person is not normally accepted as a defence in law (*Style Manual* 1994, 12.28)—although, in some jurisdictions, it is accepted that statements can sometimes be made in a jocular manner and have merely injured someone's pride rather than their reputation (Watterson 1995b, p. 52). Furthermore, even if the writer and publisher could show that 'all reasonable care was taken in checking the material to avoid defamatory content', in law this would still not matter (Watterson 1995a, p. 25).

In England, however, under the *Defamation Act*

' "innocent disseminators" such as printers, distributors and broadcasters' may successfully defend a libel suit if they can show 'they took reasonable care and had no reason to believe what they were handling contained a libel' (Whitaker 2003, p. 653). Indeed, prosecution of such entities are rare on account of provisions contained in the *Defamation Act 1996* (effective 2000) (Whitaker 2003).

For a defamation action to succeed, 'the plaintiff must prove that he or she was the person defamed by the statement' (Watterson 1995a, p. 27; Whitaker 2003). Once proved, damages and legal costs can be awarded to a plaintiff, even though no significant damage may have been caused to his or her reputation, career or prosperity (Watterson 1995b, p. 32; Whitaker 2003, p. 653). Proving defamation and achieving a successful outcome, however, can be a difficult and expensive process for a plaintiff and may result in the action being dropped or pursued via a less expensive conciliation process.

Defending a defamation claim can also be a difficult and expensive process for the defendant. Nevertheless, there are five grounds (albeit, limited) upon which the publication of defamatory material can be defended successfully:

- *Public interest*: if the truth of the allegation can be sustained and the publication of the truth was 'in the public interest' or justified 'for the public benefit'.
- *Absolute privilege*: as in the case of statements made and recorded in the course of parliamentary or judicial proceedings (recall the number of times that politicians challenge their opponents to repeat their

defamatory statements made *in* Parliament outside of the Parliament house).

- *Qualified privilege*: as in the case of publication of fair and accurate reports that have been made in good faith and with proper motive, that is, if the material has been published 'in furtherance of a legal, social or moral duty to a person who has a corresponding duty of interest to receive the information' (for example, making fair reports on parliamentary or judicial proceedings)(*Style Manual* 1995, 12.31; Whitaker 2003, p. 657). Note: a person also has a qualified privilege to reply to an attack on their character, reputation or business (Watterson 1995b, p. 36).

- *Fair comment*: if the opinions expressed were honestly held, the defamatory statements are based on facts, and/or the facts disclosed are already well known and accepted by the public, this defence is also regarded as 'one of the essential elements that go to make up our freedom of speech' (Lord Denning MR, quoted in Watterson 1995b, p. 41).

- *Consent*: where it can be shown that the plaintiff assented and authorised the publication of the material complained of (Watterson 1995b, p. 52).

For a broader discussion of these defences, see *Style Manual* 1994, 12.29–12.34; Watterson 1995b, pp. 32–7; Whitaker 2003.

There are two main reasons why a plaintiff might take legal action for defamation:

- to restore his or her reputation (that is, 'to clear one's name') insofar as this is possible

- to receive compensation for the injuries or harm done to his or her reputation, career or prosperity.

The outcome of any defamation action will depend on the following considerations:

- the nature of the defamatory material
- the circumstances in which the material was published
- the degree to which a person might feel psychogenic distress (for example: stress, depression, loss of confidence, loss of self-esteem, etc.) in relation to their loss of reputation, career or prosperity
- financial losses suffered or likely to be suffered (for example as a result of a loss of career prospects)
- whether a retraction was published by the defendant
- whether there were any mitigating circumstances (for example, the plaintiff already had 'a generally bad reputation') (Watterson 1995b, p. 53; Whitaker 2003).

MEMBERSHIP OF WRITERS' GROUPS AND ASSOCIATIONS

While there are many different writers' associations, fellowships and organisations that provide support to both novice and expert writers, interestingly, many academics and health professionals do not join these groups.

Whether or not you should become a member of a writers' group is a matter of personal choice. Membership does, however, confer certain benefits and for this reason I recommend it. Depending on the nature and purpose of a writers' association or organisation, benefits can include an opportunity to:

- meet, interact and network with other writers
- receive newsletters, journals and magazines relevant to writing, publishing and book selling
- receive notification of writing awards
- receive information on and keep abreast of changes to copyright laws
- receive information and keep abreast of taxation laws relevant to the payment and receipt of royalties
- attend seminars on writing and publishing
- access subsidised legal advice on publishing contracts and copyright issues (including the controversial issue of digital and electronic publishing)
- purchase books on writing for publication at discounted prices.

To locate a writers' group or organisation appropriate to your interests and geographical location, check your local writing guides. These generally contain lists of organisations and groups and their contact details.

In Australia, the UK, New Zealand and elsewhere, there are a number of professional bodies for writers that you should consider becoming a member of (depending on where you are located as a writer):

Australian Context
1. Australian Society of Authors
   PO Box 1566
   Strawberry Hills
   Sydney NSW 2012
   Tel: (02) 9318 0877
   Fax: (02) 9318 0530
   Website: <http://www.asauthors.org>

2. Fellowship of Australian Writers (FAW)
   FAW is Australia's oldest and largest writing organisation with branches in all Australian states and territories (refer to Rhonda Whitton's *The Australian Writer's Marketplace* or to your local telephone directory for contact details).

3. If you are a published author receiving royalties and/or entitled to receive statutory licensing fees:
   Copyright Agency Limited (CAL)
   Level 19, 157 Liverpool Street
   Sydney NSW 2000
   Tel: (02) 9394 7600
   Fax: (02) 9394 7601
   Website: <http://www.copyright.com.au>

The UK Context

1. The Society of Authors
   84 Drayton Gardens
   London SW10 95B
   Tel: 020 7373 6642
   Fax: 020 7373 5768
   Website: <www.societyofauthors.org>

2. The Writers' Guild of Great Britain
   430 Edgware Road
   London W2 1EH
   Tel: 020 7723 8074
   Fax: 020 7706 2413
   Website: <www.writersguild.org.uk>

3. The Copyright Licensing Agency Ltd (CLA)
   90 Tottenham Court Road
   London W1T 4LP

Tel: 020 7631 5555
Fax: 020 7631 5500
Website: <www.cla.w.uk>

CBC House
24 Canning Street,
Edinburgh EH3 8E9
Tel: 0131 272 2711
Fax: 0131 272 2811

4. The Authors' Licensing and Collecting Society Ltd
   (ALCS)
   Marlborough Court
   14–18 Holborn
   London EC1N 2LE
   Tel: 020 7395 0600
   Fax: 020 7395 0660
   Website: <www.alcs.co.uk>

The New Zealand Context

1. New Zealand Society of Authors (PEN NZ Inc.)
   PO Box 67–013
   Mt Eden
   Auckland
   Tel/Fax: 09 630 8077
   Website: <www.arachna.co.nz/nzsa>
2. New Zealand Writers' Guild
   Level 1, 33 College Hill
   Ponsonby
   Auckland 1001
   Tel: 09 373 2960
   Fax: 09 373 2961
   Website: <www.wga.org/iawg>

3. Copyright Licensing Ltd
   26 Kilham Avenue
   Northcote
   Auckland 1309
   Tel: 09 480 2711
   Fax: 09 480 1130
   Website: <www.copyright.co.nz>
4. Copyright Council of NZ
   PO Box 36 477
   Northcote
   Auckland 1309
   Tel: 09 480 2711
   Fax: 09 480 1130
   Website: <www.copyright.org.nz>

SUMMARY

The conduct of writing and publishing, like any professional activity, is bound by strict professional, ethical and legal standards. Writers have an obligation to ensure that they are well informed about these standards and use them effectively to inform and guide their conduct and career as writers. Writers need to be particularly aware of their rights and responsibilities in regard to:

- academic freedom
- academic integrity (and the principles of ethical writing)
- publishing contracts
- copyright
- defamation.

EXERCISES

1. Visit either the Australian Society of Authors website at <http://www.asauthors.org>, the Society of Authors (UK) website at <www.society ofauthors.org>, or the New Zealand Society of Authors website at <www.arachna.co.nz/nzsa> and consider the information provided on checking publishing contracts and on member-ship.

2. Visit the following websites to consider the infor-mation on copyright, and the rights and respon-sibilities of authors in regard to copyright issues:

   • Australian Copyright Council:
     <http://www.copyright.org.au/page3.htm>
   • Commonwealth Attorney-Generals' Depart-ment: <http://www.law.gov.au>. Locate details about and order a booklet called *Copyright Law in Australia: A short guide*.
   • Australian Copyright Agency (CAL):
     <http://www.copyright.com.au>
   • Copyright Licensing Agency Ltd (CLA) UK:
     <http://www.cla.co.uk>
   • Authors' Licensing and Collecting Society Limited (ALCS) UK:
     <http://www.alcs.co.uk>
   • Copyright Licensing Ltd (New Zealand)
     <http://www.copyright.co.nz>
   • Copyright Council of New Zealand
     <http://www.copyright.org.nz>

POSTSCRIPT: WHY I WRITE

In a seminar I once conducted at Auckland University of Technology, I was challenged to reveal why I wanted to write. My response was twofold. First I explained that my reason for wanting to write related to my mission as a writer:

> In my case, my mission was very clear: to make philosophical ethics accessible to nurses and to make nursing ethics visible in mainstream discourses on bioethics, health care ethics and professional ethics. I also wanted to make nursing ethics visible in the broader political arena (at the time I started out on my mission, nursing ethics wasn't even regarded as a legitimate concept) and to ensure that the ethical issues experienced by nurses were given the attention they deserved—were legitimated. I realised very early that to achieve these outcomes, I had to publish. And I just knew that what I had to do was to publish a *book*—that publishing articles would not be enough. I was correct about this. The rest is history (Auckland University of Technology Seminar, 24 November 2000).

The book that I wrote was titled *Bioethics: A nursing perspective* (first published in 1989). It was the first definitive nursing ethics text to be written from an Australian/New Zealand perspective. It quickly emerged, and continues to be, a leading text in its field both in Australia and overseas. I am currently preparing a fourth edition of the work; its expected publication date in 2004 will mark its sixteenth year of being in print as a commercially published work. My publisher has advised me recently that inquiries have been received from Japan and India in regard to making translations of the work for nurses in those countries. It has also gone online as a text in the United States.

My second reason for writing was, and remains, more personal. I disclosed the following to the seminar participants:

> Writing for me is *freedom*. When I write, I feel completely free—free of unwanted criticism, free of censure, free of the day-to-day constraints and pressures of the job. I can choose what I write, when I will write, where I will write (mostly in my home study) and with whom (if anyone) I will share what I have written. Writing also enables me to be creative—to craft words and sentences, and ultimately to craft stories and ideas. But most of all, writing provides me with an opportunity to make a difference—to question and call into question the assumptions of the taken-for-granted world around me. Sometimes what I write causes me deep anxiety and I pace at night wondering if I should publish what I have written—being ever mindful of the maxim, that: 'The printed word can be a most unforgiving thing'. Other times,

what I write calms me and I can prepare for the next day and its round of anxiety-provoking challenges. I have worked hard for this freedom and I am not about to let it go (Auckland University of Technology Seminar, 24 November, 2000).

I hope that in embarking on and developing your own writing career you not only find the freedom to write but in writing, find freedom—namely to think, to question, to challenge and *to be*. I also hope that once you have mastered the art and craft of writing well, you will discover and experience that writing good journal articles, good book chapters and good books can be just as satis-fying and just as informative, sometimes even more so, as reading them.

BIBLIOGRAPHY

A Concise Dictionary of Law, 1990. 2nd edn, ed. E. Martin, Oxford University Press, Oxford

Arblaster, A. 1974. *Academic Freedom*, Penguin Education, Harmondsworth, Middlesex

Archer, R. 1991. 'Explorations' in *Tall Poppies Too*, ed. S. Mitchell, Penguin Books, Ringwood, VIC, pp. 28–43

Arias, J. 2001. *Paulo Coelho: Confessions of a pilgrim*, Harper-Collins, Sydney

Armstrong, M., Lindsay, D., and Watterson, R. 1995. *Media Law in Australia,* 3rd edn, Oxford University Press, Melbourne

Australian Copyright Council. 2002a. *Information Sheet G10: An introduction to copyright in Australia*, Australian Copyright Council, Sydney

—— *Information Sheet G23: Duration of copyright protection*, Australian Copyright Council, Sydney

—— 2001a. *Information Sheet G43: Moral rights*, Australian Copyright Council, Sydney

—— 2001b. *Information Sheet G13: Writers & copyright*, Australian Copyright Council, Sydney

—— 2001c. *Information Sheet G34: Quotes & extracts: Copyright obligations*, Australian Copyright Council, Sydney

—— 2001d. *Information Sheet G15: Legal protection of ideas*, Australian Copyright Council, Sydney

—— 2001e. *Information Sheet G24: Assigning & licensing rights*, Australian Copyright Council, Sydney

—— 2001f. *Information Sheet G1: Australian Copyright Council: Who we are; what we do*, Australian Copyright Council, Sydney

Australian Nurses Journal. 1982. 'Another professional dimension within the grasp of everyone: writing for the "Journal" ', *Australian Nurses Journal*, vol. 11, no. 8, pp. 23–7

Barendt, E. Lustgarten, L., Norrie, K and Stephensen, H. 1997. *Libel and the Media: The chilling effect*, Clarendon Press, Oxford

Baverstock, A. 2002. *One Step Ahead: Publicity, newsletters and press releases*, Oxford University Press, Oxford

Beauchamp, T. and Childress, J. 2001. *Principles of Biomedical Ethics,* 5th edn, Oxford University Press, New York

Benhabib, S. 1992. *Situating the Self: Gender, community and postmodernism in contemporary ethics*, Polity Press, Cambridge, UK

Blythe, W. (ed.) 1998. *Why I Write: Thoughts on the craft of fiction*, Little, Brown and Company, Boston

Bradbury, R. 1990. *Zen in the Art of Writing*, Bantam Books, New York

Bryant, R. 1999. *Anybody Can Write: A Playful approach: Ideas for the aspiring writer, the beginner, the blocked writer*. New World Library, Novato, California

Caplan, A. (ed). 1992. *When Medicine Went Mad: Bioethics and the holocaust*, Humana Press, Totowa, New Jersey

Carroll, L. 1962. *Alice's Adventures in Wonderland* and *Through the Looking Glass*, Puffin Books, Harmondsworth, Middlesex [combined volume first published by Puffin Books, 1962]

Cixous, H. 1993. *Three Steps on the Ladder of Writing*, Columbia University Press, New York

Coelho, P. 1999. *Veronika Decides to Die*, HarperCollins, Sydney

—— 1988. *The Illustrated Alchemist: A fable about following your dream*, HarperFlamingo, New York

Collins English Dictionary. 1995. HarperCollins, Sydney

Conroy, P. 1998. 'Stories' in *Why I Write: Thoughts on the craft of fiction*, ed. W. Blythe, Little, Brown and Company, Boston, pp. 47–60

Copyright Act 1968

Copyright Amendment (Moral Rights) Act 2000

Copyright, Designs and Patents Act 1988 (UK).

Day, M. 1993. *The Art of Self-promotion: Successful promotion by writers*, Allen & Unwin in association with the Australia Council, Sydney

DeSalvo, L. 1999. *Writing as a Way of Healing: How telling our stories transforms our lives*, The Women's Press, London

Dudgeon, P. 2001. *Breaking Out of the Box: The biography of Edward De Bono*, Hodder Headline, London

Dunn, I. 1999. *The Writer's Guide: A companion to writing for pleasure or publication*, Allen & Unwin, Sydney

Edelstein, S. 1999. *100 Things Every Writer Needs to Know*, Perigee, The Berkley Publishing Group, New York

Edgerton, S. 1988. 'Philosophical analysis' in *Paths to Knowledge: Innovative research methods for nursing*, ed. B. Sarter, National League for Nursing Press, New York, pp. 169–82

Elbow, P. 1998. *Writing with Power: Techniques for mastering the writing process*, 2nd edn, Oxford University Press, New York

Emmet, L. 1968. *Learning to Philosophize*, Penguin Books, Harmondsworth, Middlesex

Fishman, R. 2000. *Creative Wisdom for Writers*, Allen & Unwin, Sydney

Freire, P. 1996. *Pedagogy of the Oppressed*, Penguin Books, Harmondsworth, Middlesex (revised edition; first published by the Continuum Publishing Company, 1970)

—— 1972. *Cultural Action for Freedom*, Penguin Books, Harmondsworth, Middlesex

Hester, M. 1992. *Lewd Women and Wicked Witches: A study of the dynamics of male domination*, Routledge, London

His Holiness the Dalai Lama and Cutler, H. 1998. *The Art of Happiness: A handbook for living*, Hodder, Sydney

Hoffmann, A. 1999. *Research for Writers*, 6th edn, A & C Black, London

Holloway, R. 2002. *On Forgiveness: How can we forgive the unforgivable?*, Canongate Books, Edinburgh

Holmes, M. 1969. *Writing the Creative Article,* The Writer, Inc., Boston.

hooks, b. 1999. *Remembered Rapture: The writer at work*, Henry Holt and Company, New York

Hubbard v. Vospers. 1972. 1 All ER 1023

International Council of Nurses. 1999. *Guidebook for Nurse Futurists: Future oriented planning for individuals, groups and associations*, International Council of Nurses, Geneva

Jacks, L. 2002. in *Hope Happens*, ed. C. DeVrye, Everest Press, Sydney

James, P. 1999. 'The slow death of public debate: Universities are joining the corporate world in stifling discussion', *The Age*, 4 May, p. 15

Johnstone, M-J. 2002. 'Imagining the future: Challenges and opportunities facing the nursing profession', Paper presented at the Cabrini Health Futures Symposium, The Cabrini Institute, Cabrini Hospital, Melbourne, 6 June

—— 2001. 'Stigma, social justice and the rights of the

mentally ill: Challenging the status quo', *Australian and New Zealand Journal of Mental Health Nursing*, vol. 10, pp. 200–9

—— 1999a. *Bioethics: A nursing perspective*, 3rd edn, Harcourt Australia, Sydney

—— 1999b. *Reporting Child Abuse: Ethical issues for the nursing profession and nurse regulating authorities*, Report to the Nurses Board of Victoria, Melbourne

—— 1994. *Nursing and the Injustices of the Law*, W.B. Saunders/ Bailliere Tindall, Sydney

Johnstone, M-J and Kanitsaki, O. 1991. 'Some moral implications of cultural and linguistic diversity in health care', *Bioethics News*, vol. 10, no. 2, pp. 22–32

Jordon, R. 2000. 'Put up or shut up' in *Nine Winning Habits of Successful Authors: Tips, tales and inspiration from 44 popular novelists*, ed. R. McAlpine, CC Press, Wellington, pp. 17–23

Kanitsaki, O. 2002. 'Mental health, culture and spirituality: Implications for the effective psychotherapeutic care of Australia's aging immigrant population', *Journal of Religious Gerontology*, vol. 13, no. 3/4, pp. 17–37

—— 2000. 'Diverse cultural care: A critical approach to care and caring' in *Potter and Perry's Fundamentals of Nursing*, eds C. Taylor and J. Crisp, Harcourt Australia, Sydney, pp. 114–37

—— 1999. 'Transcultural issues and innovations' in *Nursing Older People: Issues and innovations*, eds R. Nay and S. Garratt, MacLennan + Petty, Sydney, pp. 78–98

—— 1998. 'Palliative care and cultural diversity' in *Palliative Care: Explorations and challenges*, eds J. Parker and S. Aranda, MacLennan + Petty, Sydney, pp. 32–45

—— 1996a. 'Transcultural nursing in acute/chronic institutional care' in *Transcultural Nursing*, eds A. Omery and E. Cameron-Traub, Royal College of Nursing, Australia, Canberra, pp. 85–94

—— 1996b. 'Euthanasia in a multicultural society' in *The Politics of Euthanasia: A nursing response*, ed. M-J. Johnstone, Royal College of Nursing, Australia, Canberra, pp. 75–96

—— 1994. 'Cultural and linguistic diversity' in *Critical Care Nursing: Australian perspectives,* eds J. Romanini and J. Daly, W.B. Saunders/Bailliere Tindall, Sydney, pp. 94–125

—— 1993. 'Transcultural human care: Its challenge to and critique of professional nursing care' in *A Global Agenda for Caring*, ed. D. Gaut, National League for Nursing Press, New York, pp. 19–45

—— 1992. *Transcultural Nursing: An introductory teaching package for nurse lecturers and teachers*, La Trobe University, Melbourne

—— 1990. 'Dignifying difference: Multicultural health care'. Interview by P. Romios in *The Healthsharing Reader: Women speak about health*, eds Healthsharing Women, Pandora, Sydney, pp. 13–19

—— 1989. 'Crosscultural sensitivity in palliative care' in *The Creative Options of Palliative Care*, eds P. Hodder and A. Turney, Pandora, Sydney, pp. 68–71

—— 1988. 'Transcultural nursing: Challenge to change', *Australian Journal of Advanced Nursing*, vol. 5, no. 3, pp. 4–11

—— 1983. 'Acculturation: A new dimension in nursing', *Australian Nurses Journal*, vol. 12, no. 5, pp. 42–5, 53

Kehoe, J. 1998. *Money, Success & You*, Zoetic Inc., Vancouver, BC

—— 1997. *Mind Power into the 21st Century*, Zoetic Inc., Vancouver, BC

King, M. L. 1963. 'I have a dream' <http://web66. coled.umn.edu/new/MLK/MLK.html>

King, S. 2000. *On Writing: A memoir*, Hodder & Stoughton, London

Komesaroff, P. 1999. 'The value of views we may dislike', *The Age*, 4 May, p. 15

Krupa, G. 1982. *Situational Writing*, Wadsworth Publishing Company, Belmont, CA

Legat, M. 2003a. Publishing agreements. In *Writers' & Artists' Yearbook 2003*, A & C Black, London pp. 617–620

—— 2003b. Copyright questions. In *Writers' & Artists' Yearbook 2003*, A & C Black, London pp. 627–628

Levoy, G. 1997. *Callings: Findings and following an authentic life*, Thorsons, an imprint of HarperCollins, London

Lifton, R. Jay. 1986. *The Nazi Doctors: A study of the psychology of evil*, Macmillan, London

Longknife, A. and Sullivan, K. 2002. *The Art of Styling Sentences: 20 Patterns for success,* 4th edn, Barron's Educational Series, New York

Lopate, P. 1994. *The Art of the Personal Essay: An anthology from the classical era to the present*, Anchor Books, New York

McAlpine, R. 2000a. 'Develop the will to write' in *Nine Winning Habits of Successful Authors: Tips, tales and inspiration from 44 popular novelists*, ed. R. McAlpine, CC Press, Wellington, pp. 9–11

—— 2000b. 'Be professional' in *Nine Winning Habits of Successful Authors: Tips, tales and inspiration from 44 popular novelists*, ed. R. McAlpine, CC Press, Wellington, pp. 63–5

McCalman, J. 2000. 'The threat to the truth: Universities whose work cannot be trusted are worthless', *The Age*, 1 March, p. 17

McConnell, E and Paech, M. 1993. 'Trends in scholarly nursing literature', *Australian Journal of Advanced Nursing*, vol. 11, no. 2, pp. 28–32

McFarland-Icke, B. 1999. *Nurses in Nazi Germany: Moral choice in history*, Princeton University Press, Princeton, New Jersey

McPhee, H. 2002. 'Where are the writers to prick our collective conscience?' *The Age*, 30 August, p. 13

Madden, J. 2001. 'Work at home uproar', *The Australian*, 14 November, p. 26

Major, L. 2001. 'Academics demand right to speak', *The Age*, 8 November, p. 13

Manser, M. and Curtis, S. 2002. *The Penguin Writer's Manual*, Penguin Books, London

Marchiori, D., Meeker, W., Hawk, C. and Long, C. 1998. 'Research productivity of chiropractic college faculty' (World Federation of Chiropractic Prize-Winning Paper: Second Prize), *Journal of Manipulative and Physiological Therapeutics*, vol. 21, no. 1, pp. 8–13

Martin, P. and Birnbrauer, J. 1996. 'Introduction to clinical psychology' in *Clinical Psychology: Profession and practice*, eds P. Martin and J. Birnbrauer, Macmillan Education Australia, Melbourne, pp. 3–20

Maskell, V. and Perry, G. 1999. *Write to Publish: Writing feature articles for magazines, newspapers, and corporate and community publications*, Allen & Unwin, Sydney

Michaels, A. 2003. British Copyright Law. In *Writers' & Artists' Yearbook 2003*, A & C Black, London, pp. 629–638

Minow, M. 1990. *Making all the Difference: Inclusion, exclusion, and American law*, Cornell University Press, Ithaca, New York

Mitchell, E. 2000. *Self-publishing Made Simple: The ultimate Australian guide*, Hardie Grant Books, Melbourne

Mitchell, S. 2000. *Be Bold! And Discover the Power of Praise*, Simon & Schuster, Sydney

Nadelson, C. and Notman, M. 1978. 'Women as health professionals' in *Enclyclopedia of Bioethics*, ed. W.T. Reich, The Free Press, New York, pp. 1713–20

Nagel, T. 1987. *What Does it all Mean? A very short introduction to philosophy*, Oxford University Press, New York

Nielsen, K. 1987. 'Can there be progress in philosophy?' *Metaphilosophy*, vol. 18, no. 1, pp. 1–30

O'Neill, G. 1991. 'Academic hits "abuse" of university system', *The Age*, 3 October, p. 13

Page, S. 1998. *How to Get Published and Make a Lot of Money!* Piatkus, London

Rafferty, A., Traynor, M., and Lewison, G. 2000. *Measuring the Outputs of Nursing R&D: A third working paper*, Centre for Policy in Nursing Research, London School of Hygiene & Tropical Medicine, London

Rankin, E. 2001. *The Work of Writing: Insights and strategies for academics and professionals*, Jossey-Bass, San Francisco

Rich, A. 1979. *On Lies, Secrets and Silence: Selected prose 1966–1978*, Virago Press, London

Roberts, J., Mitchell, B. and Zubrinich, R. (eds.) 2002. *Writers on Writing*, Penguin Books, Melbourne

Roberts, K. 1997. 'Nurse-academics' scholarly output', *Australian Journal of Advanced Nursing*, vol. 14, no. 3, pp. 5–14

—— 1996. 'A snap shot of Australian nursing scholarship 1993–1994', *Collegian*, vol. 3, no. 1, pp. 4–10

Roberts, K. and Turnbull, B. 2002/2003. 'Scholarly productivity: Are nurse academics catching up?' *Australian Journal of Advanced Nursing*, vol. 20, no. 2, pp. 8–14

Roberts, P. (ed). 1999. *Paulo Freire, Politics and Pedagogy: Reflections from Aotearoa–New Zealand*, Dunmore Press, Palmerston North

Ruggiero, V. 1995. *The Art of Thinking: A guide to critical and creative thought,* 4th edn, HarperCollinsCollege, New York

Ryan, F. 1992. *Tuberculosis: The greatest story never told*, Swift Publishers, Bromsgrove, Worcestershire

Said, E. 1994. *Representations of the Intellectual, The 1993 Reith Lectures*, Vintage Books, London

Safire, W. 1997. *Lend Me Your Ears: Great speeches in history,* revised and expanded edition, W.W. Norton & Company, New York

Seech, Z. 1997. *Writing Philosophy Papers*. Wadsworth, Belmont

Sheinin, R. 1993. 'Academic freedom and integrity and ethics in publishing', *Scholarly Publishing: A Journal for Authors & Publishers*, vol. 24 no. 4, pp. 232–47

Style Manual for Authors, Editors and Printers, 2002, 6th edn, John Wiley and Sons Australia Ltd., Sydney

Style Manual for Authors, Editors and Printers, 1994, 5th edn, AGPS, Canberra

Sullivan, J. 2001. 'Publish and be damned? Not these days: Legal actions and nervous publishers are stifling important literary debates', *The Age*, 6 April, p. 17

Szasz, T. 1994. *Cruel Compassion: Psychiatric control of society's unwanted*, John Wiley & Sons, New York

Tate, D. 1989. *Health, Hope, and Healing*, M. Evans and Company, New York

The *Age*. 2003. 'Pumped Philippoussis tames a tough Thai', The *Age* 16 January, p. 1

The New Fontana Dictionary of Modern Thought. 2000. HarperCollins, London

The New Oxford Dictionary of English. 2001. Oxford University Press, Oxford

The Times Book of Quotations. 2000. HarperCollins, Glasgow

The X-Files: 'The truth'. 2003. TV Channel 10 (Melbourne), 29 January, 8.30 p.m. (S 113523)

Thomas, S. 2000. *How to Write Health Sciences Papers, Dissertations and Theses,* Churchill Livingstone, Edinburgh

Thompson, P. 2000. *The Secrets of the Great Communicators*, ABC Enterprises, Sydney

—— 1998. *Persuading Aristotle: The timeless art of persuasion in business, negotiation and the media*, Allen & Unwin, Sydney

Tzu, Sun. 1988. *The Art of War* (trans. by T. Cleary), Shambhala, Boston, Mass

van Hooft, S., Gillam L. and Byrnes, M. 1995. *Facts and Values: An introduction to critical thinking for nurses*, MacLennan + Petty, Sydney

Walker, Dale., Campbell Reesman, Jeanne, (eds). 1999. *No Mentor but Myself: Jack London on writing and writers,* 2nd edn, Standford University Press, Standford

Watterson, R. 1995a. 'Defamation' in *Media Law in Australia,* 3rd edn, M. Armstrong, D. Lindsay and R. Watterson, Oxford University Press, Melbourne, pp. 9–30

—— 1995b. 'Defamation: Defences and remedies' in *Media Law in Australia,* 3rd edn, M. Armstrong, D. Lindsay and R. Watterson, Oxford University Press, Melbourne, pp. 31–54

Whitaker, A. 2003. Libel. In *Writers' & Artists' Yearbook 2003*, A & C Black, London, pp. 653–660.

Whitton, R. 2001. *The Australian Writer's Marketplace 2002*, 5th edn, Bookman Directories, Melbourne

Wilson, N. and Thomson, G. 1999. 'Content analysis and publication outcomes of projects by public health medical registrars', *Australian and New Zealand Journal of Public Health*, vol. 23, no. 5, pp. 541–42

Winokur, J. (ed.) 1999. *Advice to Writers*, Vintage Books, New York

Witz, A. 1992. *Professions and Patriarchy*, Routledge, London

Woolf, V. 1945. *A Room of One's Own*. Penguin Books, London

Writers' & Artists' Yearbook 2003. A & C Black, London

Zilm, G. and Entwistle, C. 2002. *The SMART Way: An introduction to writing for nurses*, 2nd edn, W.B. Saunders, Toronto

Zinsser, W. 1998. *On Writing Well: The classic guide to writing nonfiction*, 6th edn. HarperPerennial, New York

INDEX

AUTHOR CONTACT INFORMATION

If you would like Megan-Jane Johnstone to facilitate a workshop or seminar on writing for publication or to speak at a conference on the issues addressed in this book, please write to:

Professor Megan-Jane Johnstone
Department of Nursing and Midwifery
RMIT University
PO Box 71
Bundoora VIC 3083
AUSTRALIA
Ph: (03) 9925 7453
Fax: (03) 0467 1629
E-mail: <megan.johnstone@rmit.edu.au>